LIVE *Healthier*

LIVE *Happier*

WITH THE HELP OF 101+ SUGGESTIONS, FORMULAS, POEMS, MANTRAS, AND LESSONS LEARNED FROM SHORT STORIES

PRATAP C. SINGHAL, MD

973-619-2707

Winterlight Books
Shelbyville, KY USA

Live Healthier, Live Happier
By Pratap C. Singhal, MD

First Printing—April 2010
ISBN: 978-1-60047-413-2

Library of Congress Control Number: 2010925061

Printed in the U.S.A.

0 1 2

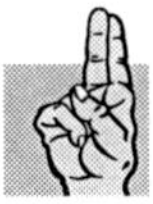

The Promise!

Of a Healthy and Happy Person

In the journey of my life I do not know
How many difficulties I will have to face,
How many obstacles I will come across,
Or how many difficult people
I will have to deal with.

But today, I promise that I will deal with
All people, situations and obstacles in a calm,
Relaxed, and composed manner
So that I can live long, and be healthy and happy.

To you:

What do you think of this promise?

I suggest you keep thinking about this idea as you go through the book. For now, just dip into the book…

Warning/Disclaimer

The focus of this book is to guide you on how to live healthier, longer, and happier. Please remember for the best results your dedication and commitment is essential on an ongoing basis. It is not a one-day affair; however, it is an achievable goal.

I have made every effort to make this book as complete and as accurate as possible. However there still may be mistakes in the content or typography. Therefore the information in this book should be considered as a general guide and not a prescription to address your specific problem(s).

The author and publisher shall have neither liability nor responsibility to any person or entity with respect to any loss or damage caused, or alleged to have been caused, directly or indirectly, by the information contained in this book. Therefore the purchaser/reader must assume full responsibility for the use of the book or the information therein.

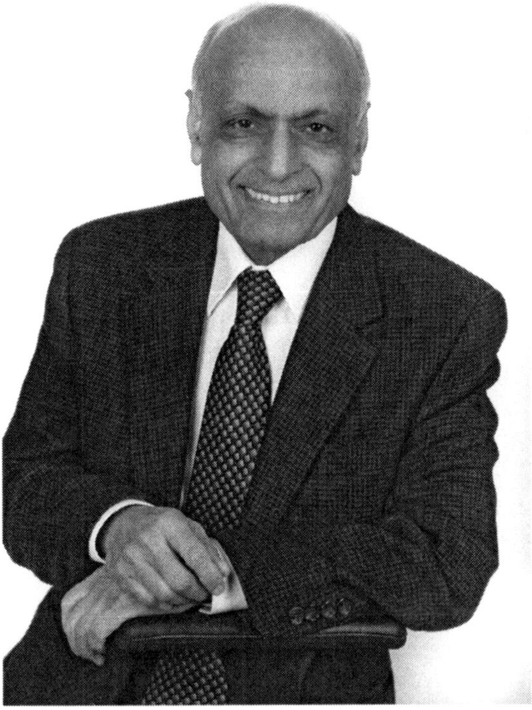

The Author

Pratap C. Singhal, MD, is a physician who practices conventional, and body mind medicine.

He firmly believes that one of our most important goals is to lead the life of mental stability and/or happiness that has a basis on being strong in the body, mind, and spirit.

He is passionate about the fact that health and happiness is within the reach of each and everyone. It is a learnable art and science that anybody can learn with training and patience. It has nothing to do with one's education, college degrees, wealth, social status, or family background.

Dr. Singhal speaks, consults, and coaches on this philosophy. For more information, go to his website, **www.livehealthierlivehappier.com**.

Acknowledgements

I take this opportunity to acknowledge and appreciate the association of those people who have made a difference in my life and have empowered me in many ways. The first and the foremost are my parents, late Mahasha Kundan lal Ji and the late Mrs. Lajwanti Ji of Dhuri, Punjab, India, whose love and wisdom will always echo in my heart and soul as long as I live. They have taught me many values of life. The one which is most worthy of mentioning is the value of love and respect for all beings, especially towards my patients. It was a God-made association.

I need to thank my wife Sushum for giving birth to three good and healthy children: Arun, Sunil, and Dhruv. They are equally blessed with their spouses: Monika, Sanchita, and Rebekka respectively. I am equally blessed with five grandchildren at the time of the publication of this book, namely, Kieran, Meera, Sonia, Sarin, and Sarina.

I would also like to acknowledge all of my brothers, sisters, and their families with whom I grew up in a cordial and loving atmosphere in the early years of my life. They are late Mahatma Prem Prakash and Mrs. Sita Devi, Mahatma Pratigya Paul and late Mrs. Sarla Devi, Mr. and Mrs. Surinder Paul and Bimla Rani, Mr. and Mrs. Raj Paul and Madhu Rani, Mr. and Mrs. Dharam Paul and Darshana Devi, Mr. and Mrs. Yog Paul and Kunu Rani. Also late sister Saraswati Devi and late Mr. Diwan Chand, sister Prakasho Devi, and late Mr. Madan Lal, and sister Pushpa Devi and Mr. Jai Lal Gupta.

I wish to express my special thank my three nephews, Mr. Vikram Singhal, Mr. Vivek Singhal and Anil Singhal, for giving me the support and help even in the odd hours of the day.

I have some special relatives who have encouraged and inspired me from time to time. They are Mr. and Mrs. Amrit Lal and Bharti Singhal and Mrs. Raj Dulari Jain.

I would like to acknowledge the association with the late Mr. Dharam Jit Jigyasu of Flushing, NY who was Vedic scholar and a practical man. He inspired me to establish an Arya Samaj/Om Temple in Belleville, N.J. (USA).

I'd like to honor two great swamis (spiritual monks) of highest caliber, namely Swami Dayanand Saraswati and Swami Vivekanand, whose teachings have influenced my life. These souls knew only how to give. I would also like to acknowledge three great yogis, namely, Anand Swami Ji, Anand Bhikshu Ji and Swami Atama Anand Ji. Meeting with these yogis was one of the fortunate experiences of my life. I have learned many of the spiritual values from them.

I will like to acknowledge some other people who have encouraged or inspired me in one way or the other. They are late Mr. and Mrs. Bansi Ram Aggraval, late Mr. Atam Parkash, Drs: Mr. and Mrs. Manikant and Jyoti Desai, Drs: Mr. and Mrs. Sankat and Manju Mandal, Mr. and Mrs. Glenn and Krista Cullen. Dr. Dinesh Nettar and Mrs. Raj Bansal, Dr. Megh Raj Goyal, Mr. and Mrs. Bobby and Rita Chatterji, Mr. and Mrs. Suresh and Prem Gupta, Mrs. Manisha Garg, Mr. and Mrs. Rajneesh and Mini Aggarwal, Mr. and Mrs. Jitenter Gupta, Mr. and Mrs. Vidya and Sudha Garg, Mr. Davinder Bansal, Mr. Sudershan Garg, Mr. and Mrs. Kamlesh and Suluxna Goyal, Mr. John Nicolas, and Mrs. Shelley Stockwell-Nicholas.

I would also like to acknowledge some of my friends with whom I have had long-term relationships from school days. These are Mr. Rup Chand Jindal, Mr. Prem Chand Singla, late Mr. Deo Raj Verma, Mr. Dharm Paul Dhir, late Dr. Girdhari Lal, Dr. Jeet Mehta, Dr. Dharam Batish, Mr. Inder Raj Singhal, and Mr. Krishan Garg. Late Mr.Yoginder Paul, Dr. Tilak Raj Girdhar and Dr. Baldev Raj Bhandari.

I am proud to be part of Clara Maass Medical Center in Belleville, NJ, where I have received support from the administration and medical staff. To name only a few of them: Mr. Thomas Biga (CEO), Dr. Keshav Shiva, Dr. Gatri Keshav, and Dr. Mehul Shah. Dr. Edward Kalmar Jr., Dr. Arthur Lester, Dr. Michael Gentile, Dr. Frank Mazzarella, Dr. Senthamarai Gandhi, Dr. Devang Gandhi, Dr. Edward S. Johnson, Dr. Joshua S. Landsman, Dr. Louis P. Allora, Dr. Philip Eichler, Dr. Wayne Caputo, Dr. Roderick Clemente, Dr. Donald Beggs, Dr. Jack Boghossain, Dr. Hemalatha Vasireddy Dr. Padmavathy Alli, Dr. Ajit Shah, Dr. Mario Criscito, Dr. Anthony Casella, Dr. Patrick Cicone, Dr. Anthony Del Gaizo, Dr. Erol Ulker, Dr. Matthew De Luca, Dr. Michael Brand, Dr. James Amato Sr., Dr. Frank Femino, Dr. Efthymios Daniskas, Dr. Jashvant Amin, Dr. Parul Amin, Dr. Neil Dello Russo, Dr. Naresh Rana,Dr. James V. Agresti, Dr. Edwin A. Amirata, Dr. Laureto Bada Jr., Dr. Hemlata Bhatia, Dr. Robert Brautigan, Dr. Edwin M. Gangemi Dr. Francis E. Cangemi, Dr. Inderpal Chadha, Dr. Eugene A. Chiappetta, Dr. Stephan Cizmar, Dr. Fiore De Vito, Dr. Srinivasa Eswarapu, Dr. John Fontanetta, Dr. Peter Gould, Dr. David J. Greifinger, Dr. Howard Groder, Dr. James A. Heimann, Dr. David Kenigsberg, Dr. James M. Orsini, Dr. Rama Reddy, Dr. Dominick A. Rubino, Dr. Jahir C. Sama, Dr. Luis Santos, Dr. Edward J. Vecchoine, Dr. Sang W. Yoo, Dr. David Zeman and many others.

I have some relatives in India who have also given me love and support. They are Mr. Pramod Singhal, Mr. Amarnath Bansal (Barnala), Professor Sunita Dhir (Director of Cultural Affairs at Panjabi University Patiala), Professor Vikram Kumar Viveki, Professor at Punjab University Chandigarh, Dr. Suresh Bansal, and Drs. Ved and Kajal Bansal.

In Arya Samaj, I received encouragement from Drs. Mr. and Mrs. Abhay and Anjuli Suda, Drs. Mr. and Mrs. Satyender and Kamlesh Khanna, Dr. Ramesh Tandon, Mr. and Mrs. Krishan and Sudesh Kapur, Dr. and Mrs. Jagdish and Punam Dang, Mr. and Mrs. Narender and Madhu Gupta, Drs: Mr. and Mrs. Hiren Gupta, Mr. Satish Sharma and Mr. Naresh Chand, Mr. and Mrs. Mahabir and Parveen Jain, Dr. Rajinder and Mrs. Jyoti Gandhi, Dr. M.G. Prasad, Dr. Baldev Achraya, Mr. Baljit Shastri, Dr. Ramesh Gupta, Mr. Vimal Velani, Mr. B. Rajpurohit, Mr. Bireder Kumar, Dr. Dev Ketu and Mr. Balraj Uppal.

I'd like to honor some Arya Samaji who are doing a great job. These are Mr. Pandit Ram Lall, Dr. Satish Prakash, Mr. Acharya Darshanand, Pandit Bharat Singh, Acharya Vedshrami, Acharya Prem Chand Shridhar, Mr. Girishi C. Khosla, Arya Pathik, Vanaprasti, Mr. Balbir Khosla, Shri Brahm Rattan Agarwal, Shri Chaman Lal Gupta, Mr. Amar Erry, Dr. Ravi Srivastava , Shri C.P.Gupta, Mr. Vikrant Ahuja, Mrs. Kamini Pahuja, Mr. Pandit Sunil Dev, Pandit Gyanender Narayan, Dr. Satish Bhatnagar and Prof. Ved Shravah.

. Special thanks to Mrs. Ritu Chopra, for her thoughtfulness and suggestions. (She is the Author of "Mastering Life, *Exploring your untapped potential to reach new heights"*

My special thanks also to Dr. Avinash Gupta and Mrs. Prem Gupta for their encouragement and support for the cause of Arya Samaj.

I also have a very special relationship with my patients. They shared their experiences with me, as I took care of their medical needs. I shall always cherish that.

I am sure I have not mentioned everyone that I should have mentioned, and I would like to apologize to those. But I can tell all those that I value your association and acquaintance.

I would like to thank Yessenia Concepcion for typing the manuscript, and to Mr. Louis Molina for his contribution.

Finally I would like to thank Susan Giffin, the editor, for her dedicated hard work.

I must thank the readers for giving me the opportunity to be part of their well being.

Sincerely,

Pratap C. Singhal, MD

Contents

B. Mental Level

C. Spiritual Level

SECTION III: METHODS & MEANS FOR A HAPPIER LIFE

SECTION IV: DOCTOR, I AM SICK!

INTRODUCTION

Please read me...

My dear friends welcome! And thank you for choosing this book.

You must have chosen this book for a strong reason. Either you are looking for ways to improve your health or you are a lover of health and happiness. Whatever the reason may be, you are correct, and your thinking is in alignment with my thinking.

Now think for a minute: If you are sick and miserable, you may have everything in abundance, e.g., wealth, college degrees, good family, and good social status, but you may not be able to enjoy life. Conversely, if you are healthy and happy, you enjoy life, and you are content with less of everything. In other words, having health and happiness is the number one priority of life, not number two. You should always keep in mind that this is a very long life.

In this reference, let me advise you that whether you live the life of health and happiness or disease and suffering, it can be your choice. I will show you how!

The story behind this book

I have been thinking for a long time as to why there is so much disease, pain, suffering, misery, and unhappiness beside all the goodness around us. We are surrounded by caring and loving parents, family, good-intentioned friends, teachers, and gurus. Every sort of information is available to us. Our scriptures have done a wonderful job in guiding us in the right direction. Even the Constitution of our country is written for freedom and happiness of all. We have a beautiful body, powerful mind, sharp intellect, and immortal soul. The sun, moon, stars, and galaxies are also for our benefit. Air, water, fire, ether, and minerals are here to nourish us. Yet we continue to suffer day after day, month after month, and year after year (even life after life, if you believe in reincarnation).

One day I was meditating, and a thought dawned on me. The thought was so beautiful, powerful, and enlightening that it brought thrill and excitement to me. It even felt like my heart was jumping up and down. Now let me share this thought with you:

Health and happiness lies within the heart and soul of each individual and not outside, and we do not need anything additional for our happiness. However, in order to make this realization come true and in order to enjoy a life of health and happiness, we need to be strong at the physical, mental, and spiritual levels. This is the focus of this book.

A strong person is always healthy, happy, and victorious in life; whereas a weak person is the victim of pain, disease, suffering, and unhappiness. There should be no doubt about it.

I can tell you that from the very beginning this book is simple and practical. No jokes and no fiction. You can read and apply the information in this book. It is that easy. I will guide you all the way through the process.

There are four sections in this book, and each one is divided into chapters. Each chapter has an objective or a mission, and at the end there is a paragraph about the benefits of that chapter. This is what makes this book useful and practical.

Imagine the positive effect on your life even if you use just one piece of information from each chapter. Of course for maximum benefit, you must make a commitment and take the responsibility for all of your acts and deeds.

To add to the practicality of the book, I have devised tests at the end of many chapters. I believe test-taking helps to clarify the subject and take you into a deeper level of understanding. Tests can also be relaxing if you are assured of not being graded or judged.

The idea of these tests is not to judge you, but to give good insight into your life. It is best that the results of the tests be kept confidential and used only for your insight and progress. These tests can be challenging, but they are also enlightening and rewarding.

I admit that I am only a student of metaphysical science and not an authority on the subject. However, the information contained in this book is correct, because I have done my own research.

Section 1

This section is devoted to the study of the self (you and me). For health and happiness, knowledge of the self is more important, more productive, and more useful that any college degree or diploma.

Section 2

This section is filled with practical information about how to become healthy and stay healthy in the body, mind, and soul.

Section 3

You must realize that the pursuit of health and happiness is an ongoing process. Here I shall guide you on how to prepare yourself to fulfill your mission of health and happiness in an ongoing manner. There is a special chapter on the art of happiness. I believe if you read this chapter with your heart and soul, it could change your life.

Section 4

This section deals with several healing methods, e.g., conventional medicine, Ayurveda, homeopathy, Natural Cure I, Natural Cure II, self-healing, fasting, and medical hypnosis.

How to use this book

I strongly suggest that you read the general section first, although it is not absolutely essential, or you can start reading any chapter that you choose. Read a chapter more than once if you feel there is a need to do so.

The uniqueness of this book is that each chapter:

1. Is complete in itself, as is everything else in the universe, including you and me.

2. Is independent; you do not need to know the information in the previous chapter, unlike a novel or science fiction.

3. Sheds new light and enlivens new hope.

4. Provides practical and useful information on that subject.

5. Relates real life examples and my experiences from which you can benefit.

I have given poetic expression to the main themes in several chapters, because I believe poetry has a more profound effect on the heart, emotion, and soul than everyday language. If you love poetry as I do, you may want to start by reading the poems.

You can bring magical transformation to your life with the help of 101+ suggestions, formulas, poems, mantras, and the lessons learned from the short stories in this book.

Writing this book has been a unique and rewarding experience for me. I saw my life evolving as I was writing it. If you read it with feeling, emotions, and commitment, it could also bring positive changes to your life. My wishes are with you.

One humble request, before I let you go on your own. You must appreciate that I have written this book from my heart and soul in order to help you. I am sure there may be some imperfections or even mistakes. Please focus on the message and ignore the negativity. This is also one of the important secrets to a happy life.

Thank you again for giving me the opportunity to be a part of your well being. Good luck!

Pratap C. Singhal, MD

I am the master of my domain

I am the master of my domain
How can I blame
To whom can I blame?
It is my life
It is my game
I am the master of my domain

When something good happens
I often claim
When results are bad
I often blame
Do not focus on the claim or the blame
It is my life
It is my game
I am the master of my domain

Neither could I make anybody change
Nor anybody could make me change
I should only focus how I could change

Or what can I do to change?
I must work with my brain
It is my life
It is my game
I am the master of my domain

I am the master and the servant
I have to face every front
This fact is well known
It is my life
It is my game
I am the master of my domain

Happiness is not in the financial freedom
I also need emotional, intellectual, and spiritual freedom
Freedom is the name of the game
It is my life
It is my game
I am the master of my domain

Gift is this life
Gift is the time
Gift is health
Gift is happiness
But I may call it by any name.
It is my life
It is my game
I am the master of my domain

Whether I chose to be healthy and happy
Or being sick and miserable
It is up to me
It is my life
It is my game
I am the master of my domain

Most people don't think and analyze
This causes problems of life
Call me Doctor, Brother Pratap or Singhal
Take my sincere advice
I tried several solutions
But came to one conclusion

I am the problem, and I am the solution
Spouse, friend, family, God, or anyone else
Cannot be blamed
It is my life
It is my game
I am the master of my domain

SECTION I

Understand & Know Yourself

This section is devoted to the understanding of you and me (the self). How do we exist at the levels of body, mind, and soul? Where do these elements reside in the body? How are they interconnected?

These answers are important, because the remainder of the book is devoted to the understanding of these elements, in making them stronger and healthier for a happier life.

Therefore, please go forward with full enthusiasm!

CHAPTER ONE

Dynamics of Health & Happiness: Slow Down/Reverse the Aging & Disease Processes

You will be amazed to know that you have the power to slow down/reverse the aging process or even the disease process at any stage of life. It does not matter whether you are a year old or ninety-nine years old. It will be easy to comprehend once you learn the dynamic nature of your body, mind, health, and happiness.

First, you do need to know that your body and mind are not fixed, but are renewed, rejuvenated, and remodeled every second from birth to death. This is the dynamic phenomenon, the phenomenon of change that governs your life.

This dynamic phenomenon offers multiple advantages over the static or fixed phenomenon. The two most important ones that you need to know are, firstly, that every tissue is kept young and fresh and, secondly, it is easy to modify these changes as they are happening, as per our new plans, desires, and needs. As you know, it is hard to change anything once it is done.

Objectives

1. To understand that our body and mind are dynamic in nature, i.e., they are constantly renewed, rejuvenated from birth until death. This process does not stop at any age.

2. Because of the changing dynamics, we can slow down or even reverse the disease process, or even slow down and reverse the aging process.

So there's hope for each and every one, even for the old, sick and miserable, thanks to the dynamic phenomenon!

Understanding the dynamic phenomenon

Let me clarify the dynamic phenomenon with some examples. Today one may be sick, weak, and miserable; and tomorrow one may get healthy, robust, and happy. The reverse could also be true. One may be healthy and happy today, and tomorrow one may become the victim of disease and unhappiness. This is what I mean by the dynamic phenomenon, the phenomenon of change.

If some sick, old, and miserable person tells me today, "I have lost my health, youth, and happiness because of my own foolish mistakes, neglect, and abuse of my body," I will smile and give him encouragement. I will tell him, "My friend, it is never too late. It does not matter if you're old, sick, or even miserable. You still have time to change. You can slow or reverse the disease process, even the aging process, but you must be willing and determined to make the commitment for your betterment."

If this same old miserable man would have made the same statement few years ago, my answer would have been quite different. I would have just sympathized with him and not offered him much hope. It is because as I am maturing in my life, getting better insight. My concept of life is changing. Today I believe differently than I believed in the past.

Normally we see young people getting old and dying. But we are not aware of how many old people are becoming younger every day by making positive changes in their life.

Many people, who at one time looked old and miserable for whatever reasons, such as poor eating habits, sedentary lifestyle or negative attitudes, have become young and happy again. Some even have conquered diseases like cancer, diabetes, and high blood pressure. It is all due to the dynamic phenomenon that governs our health and life.

You may also have heard stories of poor people becoming rich and sick people becoming healthy and robust; the uneducated becoming educated and literate; a failing student topping the class in a matter of months. These are encouraging and eye-opening stories.

Here is a short story of Lord Buddha who founded Buddhism. Once when he was a young prince in his tender years, he saw a dead body. He asked his father (the king), "Do we all have to die?" He did not like death. This incident brought a sudden awakening. He relinquished the comforts and luxuries of the palace and left home in search of immortality. Later he became a rishi (monk). What a sudden twist!

Here is another story, this one of a great Rishi Valmiki (spiritual monk). He used to be a robber (at least this is how it is believed). One day he decided to rob two saints. These saints asked him, "Do you know that you will be punished for these evil deeds?" This stunned him. These saints also asked him, "Would your family share the punishments for your deeds?" Then he tied those saints to a tree and went home to ask his family if they would share the punishments for his evil deeds. His family told him that to support the family was his problem and responsibility, and how he did it was all up to him. They did not want to be part of the punishment. This brought a sudden awakening and became the followers of those saints.

This is how inner awakening happens and life changes. Could there be such a moment in your life?

Now here is the story of a man with cancer. This man is seventy-five years old. He was diagnosed with cancer of the lungs a few years ago. At that time, he was told he had three months to live. He refused treatment and signed himself out of the hospital. He went home and cried. He sat in a chair and started counting his days.

Four weeks later suddenly something hit him. He decided: "I'm not going to be a victim of the disease." He changed his attitude toward life. He started exercising, eating healthy, and I do not know what else. I met him after three years. He's healthy, alive, and has no evidence of cancer.

You see how positive changes can change one's life? This may not apply to all cases, but this is a true story.

I can tell you another story. When I was in college, I was a good student but my English was not good. One day I met personally with my English professor and asked him what I should do. He was a wise professor. He advised me that it would be easy as long as I was willing to work hard. He suggested that I start by re-reading a middle grade English book and then a high school English book, and so on. I still remember that incident today. This applies not only to learning the English language, but also to anything and everything in life, whatever we wish to improve and advance.

Lesson: Start with the basics and then go up gradually.

Dynamics of the body

Everything in the body is on the go, like everything else in the universe. The body is not like the still water of a pond with algae and fungi, but like the fresh clean water of the stream. The body is not like the still air in a sewage pipe, but like the fresh clean air of the garden that is being refreshed every second. This is in keeping up with the dynamics of the universe.

Applying the principle of dynamics, one should be aware that all the tissues of the body are constantly being replaced by newer and younger tissues on a regular basis. At the end of every two years, the majority of the tissues are new. And at the end of every few years, the body has everything new. It is important to understand that no matter how old you are, whether you are one year old or ninety-nine years old, this remodeling process continues non-stop.

Anything that has life follows the same principle, whether it is a tiny worm or a huge elephant. (In contrast, anything that is non-living starts to deteriorate from the time it is produced, i.e., there is no auto remodeling, no auto reshaping, and no auto repairing.) It is one of the important distinctions between living versus non-living.

Take the example of our body. When we are born, we weigh approximately six to eight pounds and have a small body with beautiful skin. Every day our extremities get a little longer and our body grows; the skin stretches, and new tissues are laid. As new tissues are laid, they do so according to the body's plan to meet the new demands. This process goes on for the rest of our life. After we reach a certain age, say in the forties and fifties, we start to get old and our body starts to shrink, but our systems still continue to remodel according to the new demands. Now our body lays down tissues that are smaller in size, e.g., smaller bones, smaller muscles, smaller skin surface. This is the dynamic of the body.

Let us look at the example of our blood. It consists of plasma and cells. There are three types of cells: red blood cells, white blood cells, and platelets.

Red blood cells have a lifespan of 100 to 120 days. That means there are no red blood cells in our body that are older than 100 to 120 days. In our blood, there are red blood cells which are 1 day old, 2 days old, 3 days old, and yet others are 4 days old, and so on. Then there are some cells which are 80, 90, 100, and 120 days old. But none that are more than 120 days old. Now if you take a drop of blood from any person, it would have red blood cells of all ages, some very young (newly formed), some in the middle age (40-80) days, and some old (80-120) days.

This is the trend with all the tissues and systems of our body, not just red blood cells. Skin is being replaced every two months. Mucus membranes of the mouth are being replaced every five to seven days. Bones are replaced every six months. Even brain cells are replaced by newer cells at regular intervals. But replacement of the newer cells is basically similar to the model of the previous cells at the time of replacement, which explains why the change is not perceived. But the most fortunate fact is that we have the power to modify this process.

Do you ever wonder, although average individuals eat about one to two pounds of food per day, yet they do not gain that much weight on a daily basis? What happens to the food they eat? Where does it go?

You should have been able to guess this answer by now. It is because our body is constantly rejuvenated and renewed, and the energy that comes from the food on a daily basis goes partially to the formation of newer tissue to replace the dying and old tissue. Therefore, your weight gain is not dircctly proportional to thc amount of food you cat.

In this reference let me tell you something more. When patients go to the lab, some of them are concerned that they will be depleted of the blood they give, and they will feel weak. Just think, what about those people who donate blood on a regular basis, e.g., every two to three months?

Also understand that on a daily basis some part of our blood dies and is replaced by a newer and younger blood the same day, but this process is faster in the people who donate blood on a regular basis. This is what I mean by the dynamic nature of our body and the dynamic phenomenon. Okay so far?

Remember the dynamics of our body are in parallel with the dynamics of daily life, family dynamics, and dynamics of the universe.

Dynamics of daily life

Here is an example of the dynamics of daily life. Let's say you go to Grand Central Station in New York or any busy train station or bustling airport. What do you see? It is always full of people, men and women, children, laughing people, sad people, crying people, impatient people looking at their watches every two minutes, a constant hustle and bustle. It goes on all day and all night. You go after two hours: same thing, similar number of ladies and gents, children, impatient people, sad people, happy people, laughing people.

If you come back after ten or twenty years, you'll see the same trend. Now if you analyze, these are not the same people that you saw before. The people keep changing but the same story continues. This is like the dynamics of our body tissues.

Family dynamics

In a family, there is a grandson, a son, the father, and then the grandfather or if you are lucky great-grandfather. Now the son gets married and a new child is born into the family. Now the son becomes the father, and the father becomes the grandfather. Now the grandfather or great-grandfather dies, and the family continues. This cycle goes on. This represents the dynamics of a family, like the dynamics of body tissue. I hope now you can appreciate how our body tissues are constantly renewed.

Dynamics in the universe

Remember everything in nature is also on the go. Consider the atom, for instance. In an atom, electrons are constantly revolving around the center, which consists of neutrons and protons. Our Earth is constantly moving in several ways. It is full of vigor and energy like everything else in the universe. It is circling around the sun. The Earth also revolves around its own axis.

The seven continents are presumed to be moving. Not only this, but also the earthquakes, volcanoes, hail, storms, and tornadoes all indicate that everything in nature wants to bring changes for its own benefit. The snow is melting; the Earth is eroding inch by inch; yet new earth is formed by volcanoes in Hawaii and other places. Even the sun is not stationary. It is also revolving, making a complete circle in 24,000 years. All planets—Mercury, Venus, Mars, Jupiter, Saturn, Uranus, and Neptune—must behave in a similar trend. Galaxies are no exception. Do you know why all these changes are happening?

How easily we fail to appreciate when sitting in a garden enjoying the fresh air and the aroma of roses, while two things are happening simultaneously. Every second you are getting fresh air because air is in constant motion, and also every second the air is bringing newly emitted aroma from the roses. Roses do not emit aroma and stop; they continue to do so by their own nature and to welcome each newcomer to the garden. This is also the state of our body.

Dynamics of the body: in good health vs. poor health

In good health, the dynamics of every system are from inside out, from above below, from most important organ to least important organs. In good health, every organ eliminates its toxins outside. The nose discharges its toxins; eyes emit their discharges; ears rid ear wax; the kidneys expel urine; and the rectum evacuates solid waste. The skin perspires to get rid of its own toxins. Old skin sloughs off on a regular basis.

Now appreciate how our body fights disease. Let's say a young healthy man gets chilled in the intense cold weather and catches a chest cold. He goes home and gets some rest. The next day his chest clears up and his nose starts to run. In other words his body has thrown his chest cold to his nose, and he recovers.

One also needs to appreciate how the dynamics of good health are different from the dynamic phenomena of old age and of disease.

Dynamics of old age

As we advance in life, the same phenomenon continues, but the process, speed, and intensity of the process slows down remarkably. Toxins of the body do not come out as fast. Ear wax starts to collect. Bowel elimination takes longer, and so does the voiding of urine. The skin perspires less. The dead skin does not peel off or slough off easy. It starts to collect in places here and there in the form of growth and keratosis.

Dynamics of disease: reversal of the phenomenon

In diseased states, many phenomena get reversed. The body cannot expel its excretions. During good health, secretions from the lungs come out, but in a diseased state they start to collect in the form of phlegm, and one gets bronchitis. This is a typical disturbance of normal functioning of the system. Normally bacteria are present in the throat, rectum, urinary tract, and bladder, but they don't stick, because the body wants to keep these away and detached by a layer of thick mucus.

In the diseased state, however, the body's defenses start to fail. Mucus becomes thin, and bacteria become invasive and start to stick and attack. The result: One gets a sore throat or a urinary tract infection. Now bacteria, instead of staying detached from the mucus membrane, become attached to the body tissues and start producing toxins and making the body sick, thus breaking the phenomenon of symbiosis (helping each other). Perspiration does not come out, and sweat glands get clogged and produce cysts.

During sickness, germs and diseases want to enter deeper into the body. Disease travels from less important to more important organs (reversal of the healthy dynamics). It travels from outer tissues to inner tissues, thereby showing the weakness of the body. For example, if you get a nose cold and if you have good immunity, it will stay in your nose. But if your system is weak or you have weakened immunity, disease will travel to your sinuses and even into your lungs.

Let's say you get a bladder infection. If you have good immunity, the infection should stay in the bladder, but if you have weakened immunity then it will travel to the deeper organs, such as the kidneys or even the blood. When I see people with an infection in their kidneys or a cold settling in their chest, I know they have a lowered vitality or weakened immune system.

Dynamics of happiness

Similarly we see change in the mental attitude in many people. I had known Johnny for a long time. He used to be happy, upbeat, and pleasant. But now after his son's death, he has changed. He's always sad, depressed, and irritable.

Conversely speaking, I also know Mr. Smith, who used to be a miserable person and was very hard to deal with. All of a sudden he must have had some inner awakening, and something really must have changed him in a positive manner. Now he's always happy, smiling, and upbeat. It's a joy to be in his company.

Life is action: Swim or Drown
(Good health needs constant maintenance.)

This is the second most important principle of the dynamics of health. You know so far I have been discussing the dynamic nature of body, mind, health, and happiness. In other words, these states are transitory or temporary in nature. Therefore to maintain even the same status, you have to work at it on an ongoing basis, or things can go badly or even in reverse. To give you a simile, life is like the ocean. You are swimming in it. The moment you stop swimming, you drown!

Let me clarify this point with some examples. Let us say you go for a regular colon screening and pass the test with flying colors. Now you slack off and become lazy by resuming unhealthy eating habits. One to two years later you are diagnosed with cancer of the colon. It is because the body is in a dynamic state; in other words if you are healthy today, you may not be healthy tomorrow, unless you keep up the good work.

Perhaps you have seen some people go for a physical and pass with flying colors, and a few months later they are dead. This reinforces the same concept over and over: we have to keep up the good work all of our lives to stay healthy.

Observe another phenomenon: It is a typical example that we see on a daily basis. People want to lose weight. They go on a diet and exercise; they lose weight and are very happy. Then they slack off and return to the same unhealthy eating habits. What happens? Not only do they gain back their weight, but they also gain more weight than when they started the diet. It is because whatever we do, we need to do on a continuous and regular basis, i.e., swim or drown.

If our body is constantly changing, why we don't perceive the changes? Here are three reasons why:

1. The changes are subtle and gradual.

2. The newer tissues, which replace the older tissues, are very similar and therefore it is hard to perceive these changes. (However we can change this process.)

3. One doesn't see what one doesn't know; therefore one needs to create awareness to these changing dynamics.

Test

Before you go any further, test your knowledge to see if the message of this chapter is clear.

1. Every tissue of the body is constantly changing, rejuvenating, and remodeling. Y/N

2. This process continues from birth until death and does not stop at any age. Y/N

3. We can modify this process according to our new plans with the magical power of our minds. Y/N

4. Whatever we need to achieve, we need to be at work constantly, non-stop from birth until death. Swim or drown.

   Y/N

5. It is never too late in life, whether you are one year old or ninety-nine years old.

   Y/N

If you answered all of the questions with yes, congratulations! If not, go back and re-read the chapter.

The key message

It is possible to slow down or even reverse the aging and/or disease process at any stage of life, whether you are a year old or a hundred years old. The only thing required of you is to make a commitment and take responsibility for every act and deed.

Practical points

Using the above concept:

A. You can slow down or reverse the aging process. You can become as strong and as healthy as you were ten, twenty, or even thirty years ago.

B. You can even reverse the disease process. For instance, if you were diagnosed with a physical condition, e.g., skin condition, high blood pressure, asthma or diabetes, you should be able to rid your body of the disease or at least slow down its progression.

C. You can also achieve anything and everything that you wish to work on. For example:

If you are weak, you can become strong at any age.

If you are thin, you can gain weight.

If you are fat, you can lose weight.

If you are illiterate, you can become educated.

If you are moody and unstable, you can become calm and stable by observing silence and/or meditating on a regular basis.

If you are non-religious, you can become religious.

If you are non-spiritual, you can become spiritual.

You can learn whatever you wish to learn at any age whether it is cooking, typing, art, language, reading, computer sciences, meditation, yoga or anything else.

Enter your new plan:

____

____

Reverse the aging or disease process

The following guidelines not only help you to reverse or slow down the disease or aging process, but also improve the quality of life:

∆ Add five to ten years of life by using good breathing techniques (See Chapter 10)

∆ Meditate and observe silence for mental strength. You can add ten to fifteen years to your quality of life (See Chapters 27 & 28)

∆ Exercise for health. (You can look ten to fifteen years younger.) (Chapter 24)

∆ Increase your energy level for better health and to improve the quality of life. (See Chapter 3)

∆ Regulate your sleep schedule. (Feel like a million) (Chapter 23)

∆ Eat only for health. (Chapter 25 & 26)

∆ Miss one major meal of the day once a week. (For internal cleansing)

∆ Use the magical power of your mind to bring changes according to your plans. (Chapter 18 III)

Δ Maintain this process for continued benefits.

Scc how your lifc begins to change within weeks and months.

Mantra (Recite it on a daily basis for thirty days.)
My body and mind are dynamic (remolding and rejuvenating) in nature from birth until death. Therefore I can modify or bring changes to my body and mind according to my new plans. I can slow down or even reverse the disease or aging process.

Now here is a poetic expression of the salient message of this chapter for a deeper effect on the mind and the soul:

In the life everything is on the go
It could be fast or slow…

Life is not exempt
It is a universal fact
Take advantage of this fact
You are the magician, your body the magic
You can make anything happen
As long as it is slow or in rapid motion
In life everything is on the go
It could be fast or slow…

Life is like an ocean with mighty waves
One must continue to swim and swim
One cannot stop or slow
Or life can be over any minute
One must be clear of this fact
In life everything is on the go
It could be fast or slow…

Our body is not the pond's dirty still water
But it is the fresh flowing spring water
Whether you want to lose a pound
Or want to gain an ounce

You must be at constant work
Or it could go forward or in reverse
Because it is a dynamic process
In life everything is on the go
It can be fast or slow…

Here is the true story of a patient
Who was diagnosed with terminal cancer!
He was given three months to live
He was shocked by this verdict
And decided to live long
He went home and made new plans
Exercise, nutrition, and what else
I met him after many, many months
He is still healthy and alive
He told me it is all in the mind
You are the magician, the body the magic
You can make anything happen
As long as things are in motion
In life everything is on the go
It could be fast or slow…

Aging is not complex
Understanding is important and simple
One is only as old as one's mind
Exercise, nutrition can give extra years of life
Meditation, tranquility, and peace are bonuses of life
In life everything is on the go
It can be fast or slow …

Take my sincere advice
Call me Doctor, Brother, Pratap or Singhal
Use the power of intelligence and the mind
Be in charge and master of your life
It can turn things around in no time
In life everything is on the go
It can be fast or slow.

Now that we have studied the dynamic nature of health and life, let us turn our attention to "balance." We need to understand that balance is required at every level of life.

CHAPTER TWO

Balance in Life: The Secret to Good Health & Happiness

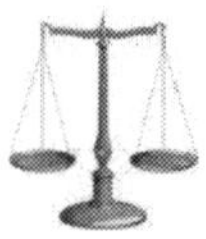

Balance in life is one of the golden secrets of achieving good health and happiness. You can also say that good health and happiness are indications of balance; whereas disease and suffering are indications of imbalance. I believe reading this chapter will enhance your ability to diagnose and even create balance in life. Are you ready?

We become amazed or even envious when we encounter a physically balanced person who is invincible; or a mentally balanced person who stays calm and collected in life's tough situations; or a spiritually balanced person who is not bothered by any situation.

We can easily appreciate the balanced personality of healthy and happy people. We can also appreciate the balance in united and happy families. Balance exists between a husband and wife, between parents and children, between love and discipline, and so on.

Of course, we all know how balance is maintained at governmental levels, whether in a city, state, or nation: Two opposite parties play an active role in maintaining such balance. In fact, the whole universe is in a state of balance. Why is Earth 93 million miles from the sun—not 92 or 94 million? Probably because at 93 million miles, the attracting forces of the sun are neutralized by the counteracting forces of Earth. We all know that the moon is a quarter million miles away from Earth—probably for the same reason: such a distance is required to counteract the two opposing forces of the Earth and moon. This is how the whole universe is set up, including the stars and galaxies.

In the universe, balance is maintained by two opposite forces counteracting each other, such as push and pull, good and bad, love and discipline, and attraction and repulsion.

Objective

Balance at the physical, mental, and spiritual levels is one of the most important ingredients of a healthier and happier life.

Definition

Let's look at how the dictionary defines it. *The Oxford Dictionary* defines *balance* as mental and emotional stability or a condition in which different elements are equal or in correct proportion; to put in a steady position.

Understanding Balance

At the health level according to Ayurveda, balance is maintained by *vata*, *pitta*, and *kapha*. According to naturopathic medicine, balance is maintained by acidity and alkalinity. In conventional medicine, doctors often try to balance the two opposite conditions. For example, if the blood pressure is too high, they bring it down; if it's too low, they bring it up. Similarly if the blood glucose is too low, they bring it up; if it's too high, they bring it down. At the mental level, depressed patients take stimulants to bring them up, while manic patients are brought down to reality.

The discipline of yoga stresses a very important point: "balance of the mind" is the secret of a healthy and happy life.

I have prepared the following list of balances and imbalances at the physical, mental, and spiritual levels for your insight and learning. I am sure you could think of additional entries to enlarge the list. Please make sure that you have fun while learning from the list. In addition, try to focus on your own imbalances as you go through the list, and how to fix them.

Physical level

1. Some people have overly dry skin; others have overly oily skin. Some people cannot perspire at all; they go to a sauna and exercise to perspire just a little. Others perspire so much that they need to change their clothes two or three times a day.

2. Some people have such a dry nose that they must carry saline mist at all times; others have a constantly runny nose and are never without a tissue.

3. Some people have very little hair or are bald, while others have hair all over their body, including on the face, nose, and forehead, making them look like a bear.

4. Some people cannot digest even the simplest of the foods while others eat like a horse—as if the food is going to run out.

5. Some people chew so slowly that you'd think they do not like the food or are already full. Others eat so quickly as if somebody will snatch their food (as most carnivorous animals do).

6. Some people are always sleepy or are not satisfied even after ten to twelve hours of sleep. Others can't sleep even ten to twelve hours in a week (because they are so restless, hyper, and nervous).

7. Some people have no desire for sex; their partners wonder if something is wrong with them and why they can't attract their partners. Others want so much sex that they drive their partners crazy.

8. Blood pressure is either too high (hypertension) or too low (hypotension); both conditions need treatment.

9. Blood sugar is either too high (diabetes) or too low (hypoglycemia); both conditions need treatment.

10. Thyroid glands are either overactive (hyperthyroidism) or under-active (hypothyroidism); both require treatment.

11. Some people walk so fast that the person with them thinks that he/she is being ignored. Meanwhile, others walk so slowly as if they are exhausted, drained, or being forced to walk.

12. Some people are so constipated that they feel lucky if they could move their bowels once every three to five days. Others have diarrhea at all times and may have to go to the toilet three to five times a day or after each meal.

13. Some people are so chilly they wear heavy clothes even during summer, making people wonder if they are sick. Other people are so hot they hardly wear any clothes, as if they want to expose themselves.

14. Some people snore so loudly that they wake up their neighbors. Others breathe so shallowly that they have to be checked to make sure they are breathing.

15. Some people drink so much water, as if there is fire in their body. Meanwhile others don't drink water at all, as if they are doing a favor by leaving some for others.

16. At parties, some people overdress, making it hard to differentiate them from the groom/bride. Other people dress carelessly, as if they were not planning to come to the party.

17. Some people will do anything to lose a pound of weight, while others who will do anything to gain an ounce. Some people say they "look at food and get fat," while others eat like a horse and don't gain an ounce.

Mental level

1. Some people speak so loudly that their neighbors can hear them. They talk as if they are giving a speech or talking to a hundred people, but in reality they are talking to only one person or even to themselves. (You must have observed that.) Others speak so softly that they need a microphone even for everyday conversations.

2. Some students study so much that even their parents have to tell them to enjoy life and relax—studying is not the only thing in life. Others don't study at all, to the point that even their friends and neighbors become concerned.

3. Some people talk incessantly without a break because they are afraid that if they stop, someone else will take over, and they will lose their chance to talk; others barely speak a sentence.

4. Some people are workaholics. Others want to be on welfare for the rest of their life, even when in the best of health—as if they are allergic to work.

5. Some people drive so fast, it feels like a comet has passed you or they are angry at you. Others drive so slowly, as if they are lost.

6. Some people talk in your face to make sure that you smell their breath, while others talk at a distance, making you wonder if they are talking to you or to themselves.

7. Some people think so much they miss their flight, lose their things, and don't know where they left their belongings. Others don't think at all and need to hire help to think about minor daily decisions.

8. Some people love their children so much they spoil them, while other parents pay so little attention to their children that the children

think something is wrong with them or their parents don't love them.

9. Some people own things and enjoy them at their will. Others are slaves to their things, neither using them for themselves, nor letting others use them.

10. Some bosses are so crazy that they give ulcers to their employees. The reverse can also be true; there are some crazy employees who give ulcers to their bosses.

11. Some people grieve over the loss of a sparrow, while others do not care for the suffering of humanity.

12. Some people will not open their purse for anything; others will spend so lavishly that they end up in bankruptcy.

Spiritual level

1. Some people have no concept of life even in the last mature days of life. Others take much interest in humanity, even during their early tender years of life.

2. Some people have so much faith (even blind faith), intense faith, that they pray several times a day and leave everything to God. Others have never seen the inside of a temple.

3. Some people believe in equal rights and respect the feelings of everyone. Others will do anything to control, rule, and abuse others; equal rights have no meaning to them.

4. Some people are not bothered by anything or any situation, while others jump out of their seat if somebody utters a wrong word.

Remarks

Do you see how understanding the game of balance and imbalance is fun? Now using your own observations and/or experiences, think of five, ten, fifteen, or more opposite situations, this exercise will help you to understand the concept of balance and imbalance in your own life.

Remember if you are healthy and happy, you are a balanced person. If you are unhealthy, unhappy, miserable, or frustrated, it may be a sign of imbalance.

How to create balance for a healthier, happier life

Remember taking the responsibility for your actions and/or the results is the first step in creating balance.

The physical level

Eat a balanced diet, and balance work with rest, exercise, and relaxation.

The mental level

Balance the mind. (See Chapter 18 III)
Balance intelligence with emotions. (See Chapter 18 II)

The spiritual level

Balance between pleasure and pain, happiness and unhappiness; and between self and others.

The key message

Creating balance can be challenging, but rewarding. I am sure you have had a good laugh reading this chapter. Now just imagine how much happiness/bliss you could get by creating balance in your life.

Mantra **(Recite it on a daily basis for thirty days.)**

I understand that having balance at the level of the body and mind can provide health, happiness, and longevity. I shall live a balanced life. I know that all greatest souls on Earth are known for their balanced personality.

Balance is the secret of everything

My friend, if you want health and happiness in life
Understand the true fact of life
Balance is the secret of everything

Balance at home or at work
In the kitchen or in the bed
Balance is the secret of everything

Whether in the ocean
On the land
In the sky
On the moon
On the stars
Or in the heaven
Balance is the secret of everything

Balance the appetite
Balance the sleep
Balance your back
Balance your emotion
Balance the ego
Balance your mind
Balance is the secret of everything

Balance the action with the reaction
Balance the love with the discipline
Balance the earning with ethics
Balance the work with rest and relaxation
Balance is the secret of everything

Neither go too high in the sky
Nor go to the bottom of the sea
Stay on the land where you really belong
Neither have the fancy for heaven
Nor feel doomed to hell
Have an insight into everything
Balance is the secret of everything

Don't be too pessimistic
Or even too optimistic
Be realistic in everything
Balance is the secret of everything

Oh! My friend, take Pratap's advice
If you want happiness in life
Keep your balance everywhere and in everything
Balance is the secret of everything

In this chapter, we have discussed the issues of balance in detail. Now we will move on to the interesting and important subject of "energy." This subject is important, because energy is the basic ingredient of each and every thing that exists in this universe from the tiniest atom to the hugest elephant, and of course that includes you and me.

So, let's begin……

CHAPTER THREE

Energy: Increase & Balance Your Energy Level

We all need and want energy, and for good reasons. Energy is good health, strength, and happiness, whereas lack of energy is disease, weakness, and unhappiness.

People do a hundred and one things to get energy, but only very few people really succeed in this mission because most of them don't know how to. In this chapter, I will discuss how to increase and balance energy.

Before we start, you should know a very important fact about energy: Energy is the basis of all creations in this universe, which includes each and every thing that you see or perceive with any of your senses. Of course this includes you and me.

You also should know that everything has several levels of existence, e.g., physical, mental, and spiritual. Since everything is energy, all of these levels exist at different frequencies and wavelengths.

This is why everything in the universe is connected and interconnected with each other, because the common denominator of everything is energy.

Before going any further, first appreciate the positive aspect of the balanced energy of a yogi, a writer, a speaker, an artist, a sculptor, and so on. You should also appreciate the negative impact of imbalanced energy, both high and low. Examples of high energy in nature are hail, tornadoes, storms, volcanoes, earthquakes, floods, and so on. In human beings, examples of high and imbalanced energy are manifested in the hyperactivity mental disorder of children or in the manic mental states of adults.

Now let us consider examples of low energy. In the desert, there is no rain and no water; there are few plants. Look at the moon or Mars; there is no life. It is all empty land. In people, look at the lack of physical energy in the form of fatigue and disease, and low mental energy in the form of depression, despair, and indecisiveness. You can appreciate the low spiritual energy in the form of selfishness, misery, and unhappiness.

Objectives

1. It is interesting to know that in the universe, energy is the basis of each and every thing.

2. Balanced energy is the sign of health and happiness. Imbalanced energy, whether low and high, is the sign of disease. And absence of energy is the sign of death.

3. We will learn how to increase and balance our energy level.

Understanding energy

Definition

According to *The Oxford Dictionary*, energy means strength and vitality. A physicist defines energy as power derived from physical or chemical resources. It derives from Greek, *energeia*, from *en* or within plus *ergon* or work. This last definition is probably better because energy works from within. Our Earth also, like other things in the universe, creates its own energy by the mechanism of rotation. The real source of a person's energy is in thc heart and soul of that person.

Attributes of energy

Since energy is the basis of everything in the universe including ourselves, therefore it becomes important to understand the energy in little details:

1. Hierarchy – As everything is made of energy, so every element exists at a different frequency level. Hence there is a hierarchy of energy, from one element to another.

2. Indestructible nature – Energy cannot be destroyed by any definition. It has at least three implications:

(a) Nothing goes to waste, even an atom. Do you realize that the life of Earth is millions of years? If we had been losing even a tiny bit of energy every day, by this time Earth would have disappeared, whereas in reality nothing or not very much has changed in so many years. Why? It is because of the indestructible nature of the energy that Earth consists of. We are also part of that energy.

(b) Everything is changing in shape and form. Do you remember the story of the chicken and the egg, which one came first?

(c) We are therefore immortal. (Later in this chapter)

3. Cause and effect – a higher (or subtler) level of energy is responsible for a lower, grosser, or physical level of creation. Spiritual energy is responsible for mental energy, and mental energy is responsible for the physical energy, and not vice versa.

4. Static or dynamic – Energy can be either manifest (or static) or un-manifest or (dynamic form). Physical objects are condensed energy. Static energy is less reactive, less available, less spiritual, and less intellectual. Whereas dynamic energy is free, it takes more space and is active or reactive, intellectually, emotionally, and spiritually.

This also applies to the medicines we take and the food we eat. When we ingest any medicine, part of the medicine gets bound to proteins in our body's tissues and thus becomes less available and less useful, whereas free available medicine is active, useful, and does its job. The food we eat is static energy and of no use as such. But after food is digested, it is converted into dynamic, usable energy.

Similarly in life, the more fixed we are in our thoughts, in our feelings, in our emotions, in our locality, the less reactive, less dynamic we are. The more flexibility, agility, and activity we have, the more energy we have.

5. Changing nature or transformation – One type of energy can be changed into other types of energy. For example heat can be changed into electricity or electricity can be changed into heat. Similarly magnetism can be changed into electricity or electricity can be changed into magnetism, and so on. Also static (matter) energy can be changed into dynamic energy and vice versa.

6. Different types of energy – Energy exists in several forms in the universe. From the physicist's point of view, energy is in the form of sound, heat, light, electricity, and magnetism. Indirectly food, water, fire, air, ether, and minerals are all energy.

At the human level, energy can be physical energy in the form of body (size and shape); mental energy in the form of intellect, thoughts, and feelings; and lastly spiritual (immortal) energy in the form of consciousness and or awareness. It is further interesting to note that in health, physical energy, mental energy, and spiritual energy are in harmony with each other but at different wavelengths and different frequencies.

7. Polarity – Energy can be neutral, for example soul, nature, and God; or it can be bipolar, as in magnetism, electricity, male and female, heat and cold, and so on.

8. Law of action based on dualities – For example, male and female, positive and negative poles of electricity, and magnetism, ups and downs, good and bad, day and night, pleasure and pain, health and disease, birth and death, and so on; these dualities are essential for action and reaction. If we combine positive and negative, there would be no action. It would be neutral. When we combine male and female, one creates an individual who it is not fit for procreation or for the continuation of the species. If we combine good and bad, it will be

nothing. If you combine day and night, it would be twilight. How depressing that could be! If there is no pain, there would be no pleasure. These dualities are not created for pain or misery, but for action and reaction, which is essential for action.

Real life examples of balance and imbalance of energy

There are two classes of people, and you are one of them. You can decide for yourself. You meet and interact with these people on a daily basis. Let us analyze and appreciate the balanced and unbalanced nature of the energy levels of these people, and how it affects their lives and of others.

Categories of people

Type A personality

1. Hurried and rushed
2. Angry
3. Impatient
4. Pushing and pulling

Type B personality

1. Relaxed
2. Works at comfortable pace
3. Pleasant and calm
4. Patient
5. Cooperative

Analyze how the first category of people is wasting a lot of energy. They are working at high gear and will burn out easily. These people will probably lead an unhappy and stressed life. Their energy level is out of balance.

Now analyze the second category. These people are saving energy and thus maintaining their energy level for longer periods of time. They will probably lead a healthier and happier life. Their energy level is better balanced. Do you think you could make use of this information for your own benefit?

Evolution of energy into life

Evolution of dynamic energy into an atom

We all know by now that dynamic energy can be changed into matter, and vice versa. If you recall the "Big Bang" theory, there was a time when the universe was nothing except dynamic energy. Then by the will of God or law of physics, a big bang happened. Everything started to move and act or react briskly. Condensation took place. The sun, Earth, moon, stars, and galaxies were created from that big bang. In other words all physical objects are the products of this phenomenon. Most likely, this phenomenon is still going on in the universe, non-stop. This did not happen only once.

The reverse phenomena are also true. Our scriptures tell us that someday everything will become desolate. There will be no more solid shapes. It will be all dynamic energy and nothing else, as it was before the big bang times.

Vedas explains the formation of the atom or the first physical structure as follows, which probably would apply to the big bang phenomena as well. According to Vedas, there are five basic and essential elements that go into the formation of any structure, including the atom. They are in this order, ether→ air→ fire→ water→ and then minerals.

What is ether? It is empty space that has divine energy and no solid or visible shape. This was before the creation of the atom.

When this ether (divine energy) comes into active motion, it becomes air in motion. When air moves with speed, it creates heat and fire. When fire becomes intense, energy melts and becomes liquid. And liquid on cooling becomes solids or minerals. Thus creation of the physical condensation or atom takes place.

Evolution of atom into life and then into human beings

The basis of the hierarchy of energy is intelligence and awareness (consciousness). In the universe everything from the most primitive element to the most advanced element is made of energy. If one analyzes the periodic table of elements, it is amazing how the progression takes place from one element to another in such a smooth gradual fashion. Similarly the level of energy is directly proportional to the degree of intelligence and awareness. In other words higher is an element in evolution; higher is its intelligence and awareness.

Let us take the very basic elements on this planet which are the minerals. They lack awareness (consciousness) and therefore are dead. These have a very basic level of intelligence and have no ability to eat, grow, or reproduce but go through the process of change and evolution, as does everything else in the universe. It is the very basic nature of energy.

Next in development are plants. These have intelligence that is higher than the minerals. They can eat, grow, and reproduce. This is a very basic level of life with very little awareness. Some plants are much more aware than other plants. There is a plant known as Lajwanti which responds to touch of the human hand. Then there are plants that are carnivores, e.g., *drosera.*

Animal life is next, with a fair amount of intelligence, the ability to eat, grow, and reproduce. The awareness level is much higher than plant life, still at an extremely low level. The intelligence and awareness level varies extremely from one animal to another, as is also the case with plants. In animals everything is prefabricated at the low intellectual level, i.e., animals work instinctively; there is no reasoning, no logic, no planning, and no goal. There is no real chance of intellectual growth. Remember animals do have some level of awareness, much higher than plants.

Animals neither can enjoy life, nor seek bliss. However animals can get sad, depressed, and even cry (just think of the depressed patient). The level of awareness of animals is very low. This is one of the big differentiating points between animals and man.

Next are human beings, which are higher in development, with a very high degree of intelligence and awareness. They can eat, grow, and reproduce. They are very conscious and aware. They have great potential for intellectual growth and awareness. They want to enjoy life and seek bliss.

Awareness is also the single most important factor which differentiates higher man from primitive man. You must have observed that some people have a very low level of awareness as to what goes on in their life, while others are extremely aware of life and the situations around them. Meditators, yogi, and spiritual masters have a much higher level of awareness; so much so that they can see the past and at times even the future.

And finally God — pure energy — has the highest degree of intelligence, highest degree of awareness, and blissfulness. (It is important to understand that we all strive for that state through mental and spiritual growth and evolution.)

Our immortal nature (Energy does not die.)

Since we are made of energy and energy cannot be destroyed, so we are immortal. Then what is death? Death is the time when the metaphysical element separates itself from the physical component of the body.

Let us go a little more in depth on this issue. As you know, our life consists of two components: the physical and the metaphysical (subtle). Let us understand what happens to the metaphysical (subtle) and the physical components. The subtle body (invisible component) consists of the mind, intellect, ego, and spirit. At the time of death, the subtle body separates from the physical body. Later on this subtle body will create a new physical body, and new life begins. (See later in this chapter.)

According to Tao's philosophy, we lose six ounces of body weight when we die; probably that is the energy of the subtle body. In other words, the subtle body must weigh six ounces, and that is the immortal energy. Vedic philosophy or theory of reincarnation has a similar point of view: the subtle body will produce another physical body. However the issue of the weight of the subtle body can be disputed.

What happens to the dead physical body? You may know that matter cannot be destroyed. So our body goes through the process of recycling. How does that happen? Well, the physical body consists of only five basic elements: ether (empty and divine space), air, fire, water, and minerals. When we cremate a body (burn it to ashes), the five elements become part of the five elements of the nature and hence nothing is destroyed. Those five elements are recycled to make another new beautiful body, starting with the birth of a new baby. In others words, the old body is transformed into the new body with those same five elements. Here the new body joins with the metaphysical (subtle) component and becomes a new life.

It is amazing to see in “Star Wars” movies how people suddenly disappear to reappear on another planet. The director should be credited with the knowledge of such creation.

Energy in relation to both good health and disease

Balanced energy is good health, while lack of energy or imbalance of energy is disease, and absence of energy means death.

Physical, mental, and spiritual energy is the cause of good physical, mental, and spiritual health respectively. In perfect health and/or happiness, physical, mental, and spiritual energy are balanced and in harmony with each other.

Think of physical energy of a child and teenager, the mental energy of a researcher, inventor, and philosopher, and the spiritual energy of a saint, seer, rishi, and yogi.

Now it is time to think and analyze what are your physical, mental and spiritual energy levels, and how to improve it. That is the purpose of this chapter. Please do not rush!

Test

1. I understand that in the universe everything is made of energy without exceptions. Y/N

2. Energy neither dies nor can be destroyed. Y/N

3. I am also made of energy. Y/N

4. Health and happiness are examples of balanced energy. Y/N

5. I need to increase and balance my energy for health and happiness. Y/N

If you have answered yes to all of the questions, congratulations! If the message is not clear, you may want to re-read the chapter.

Practical points

Since increased balance energy results in health and happiness, let us plan how you can achieve that goal.

General principles or guidelines

1. Follow the laws of nature.

2. Work as dictated by your consciousness (spirit). Remember when we work with our consciousness, we get a boost in our energy level, and when we work against our consciousness, we drain our spiritual, mental, and physical energy.

3. Work in coordination with others. When we work in coordination with others, our energy level gets a boost. On the contrary when we do the opposite, our energy level goes down.

Physical level

We can also increase our physical energy level by healthy diet, adequate rest, sleep, and exercise, and also by not wasting energy on unnecessary work; not working excessively at the cost of physical and mental rest; by the yogic technique of breathing; and by leading a balanced lifestyle.

Mental level

We can increase our mental energy by positive and inspiring thoughts (See Chapter 18 III), by keeping emotion and intellect in balance (See Chapter 18 II), by acquiring new knowledge and especially understanding the self (See Chapter 4), and by keeping ego in balance (See Chapter 18 I). We are neither heroes nor zeroes. Most importantly, balancing the mind makes us calm, focused, content, and it gives us mental strength. (See Chapter 18 III)

Spiritual level

This level corresponds with the level of awareness that can be increased by meditation and by following spiritual practices (See Chapter 22). The level of awareness can be increased by inquiry, by connecting with self and others, and by understanding the divine and eternal nature of all living beings. You can also increase your energy level by meeting well wishers and sharing your thoughts with good-intentioned people and friends.

Special esoteric techniques

With the power of special yogic techniques, you can attract or draw energy from the universe for your own benefit. The scope of this book does not allow the discussion of those techniques.

The key message

You are made of energy. You can increase and balance your energy level any time by different techniques mentioned in this book for your mental well being and happiness. Remember energy does not die. So how could *you* ever die?

Exercise: Increase energy level and heal a specific body part

1. Close your eyes.
2. Put one or both hands on the part to be healed or energized.
3. Now focus your mind on the part where you have placed your hands.
4. Stay focused on that part for the length of the exercise.
5. Visualize the part getting the energy/being healed.
6. Do it for at least three to five minutes.
7. Open your eyes.

You can do this exercise on a daily basis until the part heals. You will be amazed with the results.

Mantra (Recite it on a daily basis for thirty days.)
I am made of energy, like everything else in this universe. Energy neither dies nor can be destroyed! So how could I ever die? I can increase and balance my energy level by the techniques that I have learned in this chapter.

Energy is immortal, so is everything

Energy is the basis of everything
Neither anybody can kill
Nor can it die
Energy is immortal, so is everything

Energy is ether
Energy is air
Energy is fire
Energy is water
Energy is earth
Energy is immortal, so is everything

Energy is mineral
Energy is plant
Energy is animal
Energy is man
Energy is immortal, so is everything

Energy is the body
Energy is the mind
Energy is the spirit
Energy is immortal, so is everything

Energy is action
Energy is reaction
Energy can change shape and size
Energy is immortal, so is everything

Energy is you
Energy is me

Energy is nature
Energy is God
Energy is immortal, so is everything

What you see
What you don't see
What you will see
What you would not see
Energy is the basis of everything
Energy is immortal, so is everything

In the next chapter, we will learn that each and every thing in the universe has physical and metaphysical existence. Let us see how this applies to us, and how we can benefit from it.

CHAPTER FOUR

Who Am I? (Part I) Want Happiness? Know Yourself

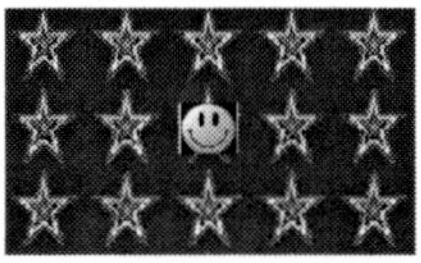

When you read and understand this chapter thoroughly, you will appreciate your divine nature. Your third eye will open, your sixth sense will get activated, and you will find peace, contentment, and happiness within yourself. You will feel different than ever before in your life.

From the time we are born, we start to question everything around us, how and why. As our curiosity grows we ask more and more questions. Then we ask a final question "Who am I?" When that question comes to our mind, all other questions look insignificant and trivial. And when it gets answered, all other questions also get answered.

Who is that "I"? The "I" is the clerk, the CEO, the businessman, the professional, the nurse, and the teacher; it is the rich and the poor, the handsome and the ugly, the humanitarian and the miser, the beggar on the street and the owner of the street. This means each and every one. Don't worry; you and I are also included in this "I."

"I" is not only the most important person in the world, but also the word "I" is most often used by everybody. Just count how many times I have used this word only in this paragraph. Try to write a paragraph or letter to a friend without the word "I." Then you will appreciate how hard it is to write anything without it. From now on just be aware when you are having a conversation with someone, how often you say or the other person uses the word "I." Remember this is the "I" that wants everything, including happiness. This is that "I" that wants to rule and control the whole universe.

Interestingly enough, the word "I" is dear to each and every one. It does not matter what language one speaks or what is one's ethnic or religious background. Now say in your heart or vocalize it: "I want to enjoy life." Say "I want to have fun." Say "I want to live happily forever." See how good it feels!

There is another special reason why this "I" is so important. How would it matter what happens to this world if I am not alive? Who cares if the world is happy or unhappy, or even if God is happy or unhappy, whether God exists or not? Equally important is the fact that understanding the self or "I" is the single most important subject of life. This we have been told time and time again by our gurus and scriptures.

So everybody should ask the question: Who am I? Did you ever ask yourself that question? Why not today? See how it can impact your life! The power of this question can be understood by the fact that people who understand or try to understand this question from their heart and soul will look at life differently than ever before.

Let us understand one more aspect: Is this "I" the hand or the brain, the heart, the body, or the mind? The more you think on this issue, the more you realize that these words do not fulfill the definition of the word

"I." Because when I say "It is my hand, my brain, or my body," that means these are mine, but not me or "I."

Now let us repeat the question one more time. "Who am I?" Am I the body? Am I the mind? Am I the soul? Or am I all three?

You have heard many times that "I" (we) have body, mind, and the spirit. You must have wondered, like me, what are these elements? Where do the mind and the spirit reside in my body? Why it is so important to understand "I" (self)?

I hope now you are ready, interested, and excited enough to dip into this chapter. Are you? Sure you are!

Objective

In order to find eternal joy, one needs to understand one's divine nature. When we say "I," we refer to the divine soul, the consciousness, not the body.

Introduction

Whenever we meet a new person, we always ask ourselves who the other person is. Not only do we ask this question to ourselves, but the person whom we meet also has the same question in his or her mind about us. Who are we?

Today let us meet the most important person on Earth and of this life: "I." Let us analyze ourselves. Let us think for a minute that we are the second person. Now let us ask who is this second person? This question "Who am I?" has been asked by many seers and spiritual researchers. These researchers have spent many years in this metaphysical study and analysis.

Here is a classical and authentic incident of Maharishi Dayanand Saraswati before he became the Maharishi (spiritual master). He was a keen person searching for spiritual knowledge and wisdom. After several years of searching, he felt frustrated and lost as to what this life is and who he is. Why are there so many miseries? One day, he knocked at the door of a great saint, Swami Virjanand. The great saint asked the question, before opening the door, “Who are you?” Swami Dayanand replied, “This is what I want to know. Who am I?” This was the turning point in the life of this great Maharishi. So you see the importance of this question “Who am I?”

I am sure if you ponder this thought seriously and long enough, it may also impact your life. Did this question ever enter your mind before? Do you recall the story of Lord Buddha? He was a young prince in his tender age when he saw a dead body, and his life changed. He started to question what life is. What is death? Who am I? What is the purpose of my life? Why is there so much misery?

Relationship of my Body Mind and Soul, among each other

Please understand that these three elements cannot function without each other. To understand this interesting relationship, let us make a deeper inquiry.

“I” exist at several levels (analysis and inquiry)

“I,” like most things living or non-living, also exist at several levels, namely physical, mental, emotional, and intellectual, and so on, or you can say physical and metaphysical levels. The best way to learn this thoroughly is to have deep analysis and inquiry.

Inquiry is the real process of deep learning. We can learn by several ways: reading, listening, watching, seeing, and doing, but the best way of learning is by inquiry. Inquiry can take one to the bottom of the ocean or the top of the mountain. Inquiry can take one to the moon or Mars.

Reading, writing, and listening could never do that. Inquiry can make the important things trivial and trivial things important.

Swami Vivekanand states: "By inquiry infinite becomes finite, and also finite becomes infinite."

To give you the real concept of body, mind, and soul, let me explain by examples of the real world. I will try to compare the body, mind, and soul concept with a sugar factory, postal service, hospital system, police department, senator's office, and banking system, and so on.

I love to compare the human body with a sugar factory. Actually you can compare the body with any system, but the reason I want to compare it with a sugar factory is because it is detailed and compact. That's how the body is; therefore it is easier to compare the two. Also I have witnessed the working of a sugar factory.

The sugar factory has three floors. On the first floor, sugar cane is brought in and crushed, juice is prepared, and pulp is thrown out. This first floor corresponds to our abdomen, where food is ingested, *rasa* and *chyle* are formed, and stool and urine are expelled.

On the second floor of the sugar factory, the juice is heated, purified, and circulated. This corresponds to our chest. Here our heart and lungs do the same job. Lungs get rid of the carbon dioxide of the blood and enrich the blood with oxygen and *prana* (energy), and then the heart moves the blood into circulation.

The third floor comprises the executive offices of engineers, accountants, chemists, supervisors, and the CEO. These executive officers use their brains to run the factory or put their heads together as to how the sugar factory could do a better job. This is the intelligence of the factory. So the third floor corresponds to our intelligence, i.e., brain and head.

Now if you analyze carefully the accountants, chemists, the supervisors, and the engineers, they report to one person who makes all of the decisions. That person is the manager or the CEO of the factory. That person is equal to our mind. Without our mind, no decision can be made.

The job of a manager is powerful, but the manager is not the owner. There is somebody higher than the mind or the manager. Managers can be fired and a new one can be hired at the will of the owner. So who is the owner?

The owner is the one who has the power to shut the factory down or fire the manager or the engineers, and so on. In our case the owner is the soul or our higher self. The soul is the owner of the heart, brain, the body, and even the mind. Now let us see if this simile of the sugar factory can be applied to the different systems in daily life.

The post office also has three components. The physical components correspond to the building, which may be like a cottage or a beautiful government structure. In any case, it corresponds to our physical body. The intellectual and emotional components are the workers who run the post office. This is also equal to our intelligence and emotions. Then there's the postmaster, who corresponds to our mind, who makes all of the decisions. Every worker reports to the postmaster. The soul of the post office is to help people keep in touch with each other by the exchange of mail and gifts.

In the post office everything can change; the building can change; the workers can change; and even the postmaster can change. But the soul or the essence of the post office will not change. Unfortunately many people think that the post office building is the post office. At least that was my impression when I was a small child and went to mail letters for my father. When people think they are the body, they are thinking like a child, as I used to think in my childhood.

A hospital has a physical component, the beautiful building which is designed for the comfort of the patient and the medical staff. Then the intellectual and emotional components are the doctors, nurses, and pharmacists who are involved in taking care of the sick. Then there is the CEO or administrator of the hospital who makes all of the critical decisions for running the hospital. He does not take care of the patients. The hospital administrator corresponds to our mind. Then there's the essence or soul of the hospital that is to help and comfort the sick.

As you can see, the hospital building can change; doctors, nurses, and pharmacists can change; and even the administrator can change. But the essence or soul of the hospital—to serve and to comfort the sick—cannot change.

Similarly a police department has a physical component. That is the building (the jail) where they lock up the criminals. Police officers are like the intelligence of the police department. The police chief is like the manager or like our mind. The soul or the essence of the police department is to protect the public and the innocent and to enforce the law. Once again, a police building can change; the police chief can change; and policemen change all of the time, but the soul or essence of the police department will not change in millions of years.

Now take the example of a senator's office; it has the physical component, the beautiful building, where the employees of the senator's office work and people come and get their problems solved. The employees of the office are equal to the intelligence and the emotional component of our body. The manager who runs the senator's office is like our mind that makes all the decisions. The essence of the senator's office is to help expedite matters for the public. The building can change; the employees can change; and even the senator can change, but the essence of the senator's office cannot change.

We can also take the example of a bank; it has a physical component. It is located in a building where the employees work. The workers are like the intelligence of the bank. The bank manager is like the administrator or like our mind. The essence of the bank is to help people with money matters, giving or receiving, depending on the needs of the people. The workers can change; the bank manager can change; or the building can change, but the soul or the essence of the bank can never change.

Now let us analyze ourselves. I have tried to impress upon you that we exist on at least three levels: body, mind, and soul. I'm not the body; the body belongs to me, but the body is not me. The body is meat and flesh, which is cremated or buried after death or after the soul leaves the body.

The body is like the post office building, bank building, hospital building, and police station, and the building of the senator's office. The building has no value without the workers, the managers, and the soul. Similarly our body has no value without its intelligence, mind, and soul. Our intelligence is like the workers in the various systems we have just studied.

The mind is equal to the manager of our life. The mind makes all the decisions, right or wrong. It is like the hospital administrator, the postmaster, the police chief, the bank manager, and so forth.

Our soul can be compared with the soul of the post office, the police department, the hospital, the banking department, and the senator's office. The soul of the post office is to help people keep in touch with each other; the soul of the hospital is to help the sick to get better; the soul of the police department is to protect the innocent and enforce the law; the soul of the bank is to help people with money, receiving or loaning, and so on.

So in summarizing the above information: "Who am I?" I will say that we are made of all three elements, as follows:

1. The physical body, the gross body, the manifest body (one element), which is dependent on mind and soul.

2. The psychic element, the subtle element, (non-visible) which consists of mind, intellect, and ego (three elements), yet dependent on soul. In other words these cannot function without the soul.

3. The soul, the subtlest of all. The eternal, the immortal. The conscious and the animating principle of life. The only independent element of life (One). That is what I am or you are.

In other words, the soul is the most essential, independent, and eternal element which needs the mind, the intelligence, the emotions, and the body to do its job. But remember the body, mind, and intelligence cannot function without the soul. But the soul works through the mind, intellect, ego, and body. So I am all three; here the soul is the owner and only independent element and hence indispensable.

Experience

I wish to narrate a true incident of my life. One time a great Swami Ji came to our Samaj and asked everybody one question: Who are you? He was very fanatical about this question, and he did not feel satisfied until everybody could answer the question. He wanted to stress upon each one of us that we are the divine soul and nothing else. We are not the body. We are not the mind. We are not the intelligence. We are the soul, the immortal.

Deeper existence of everything (multiple dimension view)

In this universe, things are much deeper than they appear. The more we analyze things deeper and deeper, the better we get into these things. That is why there are controversies on every issue, because people look at things from different angles and/or different levels of their own understanding.

Things in the universe may exist at several levels; however for the sake of study, we can divide everything into three. For example, time has three components: past, present, and future. I, you, and he/she are three. "I" above me and below me are three. Normal, good, and bad are three. Summer, winter, or changes of weather are three. Even God has three letters not only in English but also in Hindi script. Even the body can be divided into three parts: the trunk, the head, and the extremities.

Now if you analyze water, it also exists at three levels: physical, intellectual, and spiritual. In a physical form, it exists at the level of ice (solid), water (liquid), and steam (air). At the intellectual level, it contains hydrogen and oxygen. At the spiritual level, it has the power of cooling and adherence.

Similarly if you analyze fire, at the physical level it is something that produces heat. At the intellectual level, it is the burning carbon in the presence of oxygen. At the spiritual level, fire is energy and heat.

If you analyze the face of a person, it can be divided into three portions: upper third, middle third, and lower third. The upper third portion corresponds to the spiritual aspect of the person; the middle third portion corresponds to the mental aspect; and the bottom third of the face corresponds to the physical level of the person.

Similarly handwriting is analyzed at the physical, mental, and spiritual levels. Each letter of the alphabet has a bottom (physical), middle (mental), and the top (spiritual component). Furthermore, if you analyze the palm of a person, it has three components: physical, mental, and spiritual.

Let me give you few more examples because it is important to understand the concept of three levels. A movie has three components: the acting of the actors and actresses, the set for the scenes, and the directions of the director; this is the physical component of the movie. Now the thought process, the words that are being used, and the message conveyed comprise the middle or the intellectual component of the movie. Lastly the theme on which this movie is based is the soul or the essence of the movie.

Let's take another example: you go meet your son whom you have not seen for a while. For the first half hour, you will have physical contact, the superficial contact. You have a cup of tea or juice, sit down, and relax. You discuss how the driving was; how good his house looks; how nice the neighborhood is; that is the superficial contact, the initial contact.

Now you start talking a little more deeply. How is he doing in his life? What are his children doing? What school do they attend? How is his business? All these things take you to a deeper level, but not the deepest level. Lastly you talk one on one; you ask him how he is really doing. Is he happy in his life? You and he cry or laugh together. He tells you everything about his life, and you tell him about your life. This is the deepest level of contact, heart to heart, the contact: the soul contact.

Let us take the example of a business deal. First you meet, say hello, and ask how the other person is. You talk about the weather, have a cup of tea, comment on how good the other person looks, this or that is beautiful; these are superficial initial contacts. Then you start talking about the business, money, investments, how the business will go. Now you get into nitty and gritty, and that is the deeper and higher level of business. Finally you go to the contract. The final deals, the essence, the money, the sharing of responsibility; this is where business deals are made or broken.

My idea of these examples is to give you an understanding of the thick and thin of everything in this life.

The rose: the multiple facets

The rose has several components. It has a physical component, a chemical component (intellectual), and spiritual component.

The physical component of the rose consists of the collective arrangement of the colored petals, the (attractive elements), and its beauty with which it attracts all living beings, including insects. A poet describes the beauty of the rose in his imaginary emotional language. A sculpture picks up the rose and looks at it up and down, side to side. He looks at the thorns, the leaves, and the petals, and then spends some time to analyze so that he can create a reproduction of it.

A beekeeper looks at how much honey can be created from how many flowers. A lover looks at the rose and plucks it for his beloved.

Let us analyze the chemical element of the rose. A chemist analyzes the chemical element which causes the aroma to make perfume. The Ayurveda physician analyzes how this rose can be used as a medicine in preparations to cool the body. He also looks how the aroma of the rose can be used to soothe the mind. The rose also has a spiritual component. A priest or *pandit* picks up the rose for the purpose of decoration or to please God or the deity in the temple.

This may not be the most typical example of life, but it gives an idea how analysis can take us deeper and deeper into anything.

Understanding: The pain and pleasures of the body, mind, and soul

Since we live at three levels, let me clarify these with examples for better understanding.

Pain of the body, mind, and soul

The levels of pain of the physical body are superficial and short-lived. Pain of the psychic (mind, intellect, and ego) body is long-lived and more intense. Pain of the soul are very intense, very deep, and of longest duration. Of course it is true that the intensity and duration of the pain will vary based on the strength of the individual. The healthier and stronger a person is, the less likely he is going to be the victim of the pain.

Now let us take a few examples of the three levels of pain. Physical pains are body aches, diabetes, arthritis, heart disease, and so on. Mental pains are insults, restlessness, anguish, confusion, mental wandering, loss of thought process, and so on. Spiritual pains are very deep, very long-lasting; some people die with that pain.

Let me give you some concrete examples: An eighty-year-old female is diagnosed with cancer. She is suffering from pain; she moans with pain day and night. She knows it is a physical pain. She had to bear this pain until she dies. It is typical of physical pain. She has accepted disease and death, and she will die peacefully.

A thirty-year-old female was recently married but her husband died in an accident. Now she is suffers from mental pain. It is not physical pain. She gets depressed, but in a year or two she may get over it.

A thirty-five-year-old mother is diagnosed with terminal cancer. She has a six-year-old child. You cannot describe the pain of that mother. She is suffering less from physical pain, but she is tortured with the intense mental and spiritual pain. Every time she looks at the child, she cries, she weeps, she hugs her child. That is spiritual pain, intense pain. She will die more from this pain than from the disease.

On the contrary, with people who have physical pain, it disappears after death, but spiritual pain goes with the person at the time of death.

Pleasures of the body, mind, and soul

As there are three levels of pain, there are also three levels of pleasure belonging to the different elements of the body.

Physical pleasures are short-lived and easy to get. Mental pleasures are longer lasting and not so easy to acquire; it takes effort and hard work. Spiritual pleasures are longest lasting. They bring joy, happiness, and bliss, and also require devotion and sacrifice.

Physical pleasures can be compared with a rich and comfortable life. Mental pleasures belong to an honorable job, respectable position, sharp intellect, balanced mind, cooperative family, nice boss, nice spouse, and so on.

Spiritual pleasure comes with self-realization or when one can touch/reach his soul or the soul of others. When one begins to love and respect all others; when one begins to see the divinity in the self and in all others; he becomes content, peaceful, and blissful. He needs nothing more. He finds everything within the self. He has it all. That is spiritual pleasure.

Examples of people living at the level of body, mind, and soul (physical, mental, spiritual levels)

Please try to appreciate how these examples may apply to your life and how you can benefit from them.

People living at the physical level are very much concerned with their house, cars, make-up, physical body, external appearance or the materialistic elements. They are focused on the body's comfort and so on; they may be selfish in their nature. They may not be mentally strong or stable. This life is the lowest level of human life. It is like living the life of a building. Their joys and comforts are based on the materialistic items that are of temporary nature. These people are usually impatient and selfish, and in a real sense are ignorant about life matters. They don't grasp the concept of consciousness. The worst part is that these people can fall apart during the stresses and challenges of life.

People on the mental level more often think of knowledge, education, degrees, and higher status. They may be able to make good decisions and help and guide others. They may have good judgment. These people may or may not be mentally stable. It is a much better way of life than the people living at the physical level but still not the best. Their comfort, joy, and pleasure last longer than in the first category of people. The mental level people are between the two levels, physical and spiritual. These people do not make full use of their consciousness. I am sure you can do better than that. Certainly wise people can do better than that.

Wise, liberated, and enlightened people live at the spiritual level. They are very content and at peace with themselves. They have the ability to guide and help others. They enjoy helping others. They have the ability to comfort others. They see divinity in life and have a deeper understanding of life. These people are upbeat and very balanced in nature and are a joy to work with. These are very sincere people. The pleasure and joy of these people is very deep and longest lasting. The key element is that these people are content, have patience, and are full of joy because they have found everything they need.

Then lastly there are rishi, swami, and spiritual masters; they are at a much higher level of life. They understand life and its purpose. These are very advanced souls (spirit). Nothing bothers them. People travel miles to meet and see these people, to get their blessing, because they emanate peace and joy. God bless them! They are Godly people.

Simplification

1. People living at the physical level focus on their body, face, nose, belly, looks, and their appearance; this is their limit. This is their focus.

2. People at the mental level are focused on education, degrees, diplomas, and more diplomas.

3. People at the spiritual level are more focused on life, understanding life and its purpose. Why birth? Why death? What is this game of life?

Test

Test your knowledge to see if this chapter's message is clear.

1. I understand that each and every thing exists at physical and metaphysical levels. Y/N

2. I also have several levels of existence. Y/N

3. My physical level of existence is the body. Y/N

4. My metaphysical level of existence is the mind and soul. Y/N

5. My mind is the manager, not the boss. Y/N

6. My soul (consciousness) is the boss, the ultimate authority. It is the soul that is referred to as "I." Y/N

7. Now I understand that I am the combination of body, mind, and soul. Y/N

If you answered all of the questions with yes, then you are clear about this chapter. Congratulations! Or, if not, you may want to read this chapter again. Are you with me so far?

Practical points

Today you should decide at what level you want to live. You should also be clear from this discussion that everlasting joy comes only when you begin to understand self and start to question who you are. If you are not clear so far, I suggest you read this chapter again and again. Don't rush to the next chapter. Pause! Take a break! And take a day off from this book. Think and meditate on this concept before going any further.

Because I live at three levels, I also must try to analyze and understand what is meant by:

a. Food and nourishment for body, mind, and soul
b. Sleep and waking for body, mind, and soul
c. Rest and relaxation for body, mind, and soul
d. Exercises for body, mind, and soul
e. Pains and pleasures of the body, mind, and soul
f. Lastly and most importantly you need to understand that the needs of the body, mind, and soul are very different.

Remember people who stay focused only on the needs of the body will not find happiness. To find happiness one needs to focus on the needs of the soul. Soul wants peace. Soul wants happiness. Soul wants love. Soul wants compassion.

The key message

You exist at several levels, like everything else in this universe. Your most subtle and most powerful and eternal element is the soul, the spirit, the consciousness. To enjoy happiness you should work with your consciousness.

Mantra (Recite it on a daily basis for thirty days.)
I am consciousness (soul). My name is consciousness (soul). I shall work with my consciousness for my happiness.

I have expressed the key message of the chapter in poetical language. Let this message reach your heart and soul. Now enjoy the poem.

Who am I?
Understanding self is the game of its own kind
Self is good, self is bad
Self is happy and self is sad.
Understanding self is an art and science
Understanding self is the game of its own kind

I am the child, father is He
I am divine, the divine is He
I am eternal, eternal is He
He wants everyone to be kind, because He is kind
Understanding self is the game of its own kind

Understanding of Him, you, and the universe,
It looks so different and complex
But understanding the self makes things simple in time
Understanding self is the game of its own kind

Ignorant focus on the suffering and pain
Intelligent one on a better plan
One who focuses on the self
Becomes the immortal self
It all happens with time
Understanding self is the game of its own kind

How I make the body, mind, and spirit strong
For body I must exercise and eat with a plan
Mind becomes strong when one stays calm and
Focused, on the plan
The spirit has its root in being loving and kind
Understanding self is the game of its own kind

I (soul) am the center focus
Body, brain and the mind are hocus and pocus
I am not the hand, heart or the brain
Nor I am the mighty mind
I am the self and the owner of its kind
Understanding self is the game of its own kind

Body is not me, but for me
Mind is not me, but for me
Don't get lost in this complex
I can make it easy and simplex,
When one removes one's blinds
Understanding self is the game of its own kind

One who lives for the body becomes the body
One who lives for the mind becomes the mind
But one who understand the real self
Realize the immortal self
The day I realize myself
The day I liberate myself
I am the spirit and divine
Everyone else is of similar kind
Body is vehicle for me to ride
I can change it any time
Understanding self is the game of its own kind

Call me Brother, Pratap or Singhal
Take my sincere advice
If you want happiness and freedom in life
You should be thinking this all the time
Who am I, what am I?
Everything in life has a purpose and/or plan
How I can be here without a plan
What I do, what can I do
How should I do and what should I do
Why I am here, how am I here?
To understand this game, one has to
Be good and kind
Understanding self is the game of its own kind

Now, in the next chapter, "Who Am I? Part II," we dig deeper into why human beings seek happiness and bliss!

CHAPTER FIVE

Who Am I? (Part II) Why Happiness is a Must

In the previous chapter, I have tried to clarify the meaning of "Who am I?" This was important because the "I" is responsible for each and every thing in one's life. This is the "I" that wants happiness.

Now we will work on understanding why everyone wants happiness and why happiness is so important for one's life. Although many young people may not be focused on this issue, as they are busy raising children, making money, and getting an education, and so on. However, as they mature, this quest becomes more and more obvious, almost like a mission or goal in life. How one finds happiness is not the subject matter of this chapter; that will be discussed in Chapter 30.

Objective

To understand that one of the key missions in life is to lead a life of good health, freedom, and happiness. Whoever does not achieve this goal, irrespective of what else they may achieve, will not be a success in real terms.

Introduction

We all want happiness. Why not? We all need, want, and deserve it. This is also the teaching of our parents, teachers, and our scriptures. We need to know that happiness is based on total freedom, i.e., emotional, mental, intellectual, spiritual, and so on, or freedom in every aspect of life.

Definition

Happiness means wellness at the physical, mental, and spiritual levels.

Happiness: Vedic (Hindu) view of life

According to Vedic philosophy, "One must live the life of independence, freedom, and happiness." If not, then one has failed in his or her life. Freedom and happiness are based on being strong at the physical, mental, and spiritual levels.

Physical, mental, and spiritual health→wholeness →independence →freedom →happiness

Setting the goal—defining the mission

In order to achieve any goal or mission, it is important to define it first, because defining helps. See how:

<u>It leads to clarity of thought, planning, and action.</u>

People who do not define their mission in life work like machines. You know how machines work. You press one button and the machine is on, and you press it again and it is off. Similarly people without a mission get up in the morning and go to work. And at night they come home and go to sleep, and so on. There is no finish line for them. There is no end goal for them. There is no joy for them. There is no happiness for them.

<u>It means defining the expectation</u>.

Expectation and outcome are directly related to a great extent.

Helping to define the mission

This is a very important question. Take your time! Think and analyze! Don't rush! Slow down! Slowing can improve the quality! In order to define the mission, you must understand why this life has been given to you. What you are supposed to achieve in this life? You should also be clear that life is not just about living the life of a civilized animal, but also living the life of freedom, joy, and happiness.

In order to get help in defining the mission, you can reflect on the role model of the people whom you admire. Or you can learn from the gurus or spiritual masters. You can also learn from the wise people who have maintained their mental balance during all the calamities, pain, and sufferings of life. Or you can get help from the scriptures. Or you can write your own obituary, just for insight. This is nothing to feel bad about it. Remember some day, somebody will write one for you.

Cyclical nature of your life

You must be aware that in the universe everything is cyclical in nature, including your life. Let us understand what a cycle is, when it is considered complete, and what its implication is.

How do we define a cycle? Something leaves home for a purpose or a mission, and after the mission is fulfilled it goes back to its home. This is one cycle. The cycle may last one hour, one day, one year, a hundred years, or millions of years, but it is one cycle. In order to complete a cycle, anything must go back to its point of origin, i.e., home.

Why things are cyclical in nature?

1. Energy cannot be destroyed; nothing goes to waste. It just keeps changing size and shape.

2. Energy cannot stay still. Life is action; therefore everything stays in motion or in action.

3. With each subsequent repetition of a cycle, one continues to makes some progress. Each little progress eventually leads to perfection. Perfection leads to wholeness, and then freedom and happiness. This is one of the most important practical facts that *are* applicable to human life.

For a better understanding of this subject, let us study in detail the cyclical nature of water, nitrogen, and fire. Take the examples of the water cycle. The mother of the water is the ocean. Water evaporates in the form of a cloud from the ocean; it rains and quenches the thirst of the land, and returns to the ocean, its home. Here one cycle is completed. The home of the water is the ocean, so water flows impatiently downwards to reach the ocean. It flows downwards not because of gravity, but because it is restless to reach its mother, the ocean, its home, its point of the origin. Otherwise the cycle will not be complete. This is an important concept.

Let's take the nitrogen cycle. Nitrogen in the air is absorbed by plants and becomes food. We eat fruits and vegetables, and nitrogen is eliminated from the stool and urine and back to the atmosphere, air, its home, its point of the origin. Please note that the nitrogen goes up to the atmosphere and not down to the ocean.

Now let's take example of fire. The sun is the source of all fire and energy. Fire collects, gathers, or is stored in fruits, plants, and wood. When wood burns, the same stored energy comes out as fire, and this fire wants to go up. Why? It is because the home (mother) of the fire is the sun, not the Earth. Therefore fire goes up and not down.

So you see nitrogen, air, and fire: these want to return to their home or mother. Vedic philosophy states that everything is attracted to its home, its mother. Vedic philosophy does not agree with Newton's law of gravity which says that everything is attracted to Earth because of gravity. Newton's law explains that the apple falls to the ground because of gravity. According to Vedic philosophy, the apple falls to ground because the main ingredients of the apple are water and minerals, and the mother of both water and minerals is the Earth.

If the law of gravity is correct, then everything would be pulled to the Earth, including air, plants, minerals and even humans, and nothing would exist.

Now going back to the cyclical nature, let us appreciate how this applies to our human life: It is the basis of reincarnation (Vedic view of life). One is born, makes some mental and spiritual advances or progresses, and death ensues. Now one has a second birth, makes a little more mental and spiritual progress and death follows. Then one is born a third time, and the same cycle continues until one reaches perfection mentally and spiritually. Once one reaches that stage and learns to live the life of freedom and happiness, then one becomes entitled to go home (heaven, salvation). Now one cycle is completed.

The final outcome of this life

The outcome of the end of life will be determined whether or not you have fulfilled your life mission. If you have succeeded in living the life of freedom and happiness, then you have succeeded in your life and will be entitled to go home or heaven. However, if you have not succeeded in this mission, then you have to return through another birth. It is like at the end of the school or college year, the dean of the school decides which students graduate and which do not, based on their performance in school.

Do you know how you feel when you do a job well, graduate from college with honors or complete a tough project with success? What joy, pride, and happiness! You also know how you feel at the end of the day, at the end of the exam, at the end of the project if you do not succeed. What sadness and frustration! One needs to repeat the process again and again; you know how frustrating that can be. This is also applicable to life.

Why do people fail to accomplish their mission in life? Life is very busy. In a busy life they forget that they have come from the divine and need to stay divine. When, due to whatever situations or circumstances, they get attached to the mundane and materialistic things of life, they drift away from divinity. When that happens, they also become mundane. Thus, they end up in the cycle of birth>death, birth>death, and so on. But if you have lived the life of relaxation, freedom, and happiness, then you graduate from life and go to the heaven. (Vedic view of life)

Test

1. I understand that life has a purpose and a mission like everything else in the universe. Y/N

2. The mission of life is to attain freedom and happiness. Y/N

3. Freedom and happiness reside within the heart and soul of each individual. Y/N

4. To achieve this goal I need to grow mentally and spiritually. Y/N

5. My focus has been to live the life of relaxation, freedom, and happiness. Y/N

If you have answered most of the questions with yes, then congratulations! You graduate! If not, please read the chapter again.

Practical points

1. You must realize that you are eternal soul. You are free, independent, and happy. Happiness is your name.

2. The more you search the happiness within your heart and soul, the sooner you will reach your goal of life.

3. The further you go away from your heart and soul in search of happiness, the further away you will stray from your goal.

Mantra (Recite it on a daily basis for thirty days.)

My name is happiness. Happiness is my goal. I know that success in life should be measured only by the happiness and joy with which I shall lead my life, irrespective of anything else.

Let's Go Home
Let us go home
Birds fly to their nest as befalls the dusk
Grazing cattle walk to their home as the night befalls
Water goes down to the ocean to its parental home
Apple fall on the ground because Earth is its mother, not because
Newton told it so
Everybody must go home, everything must go home.

Air will not go down, nor does the fire because their home is
Above and beyond
They don't care for Newton or gravity,
They must go home and they must go home!

At the school bell rings at 3 o'clock, children go home in buses,
Car or on the foot
You see a smile because they have done a good day's work, and
Hence time to go home,
At 5 PM all workers pack up and go with a smile or
Paycheck
They have done their day's work, why should not they
Go home
Everybody must go home, everything must go home.

I belong to the supreme
And the supreme belongs to me
Either he comes to me or I must go to him
I cannot wait too long
Because there are others in a long line
Why don't I go and save time
That is my home and that is my home
We all need to go home, let us go home.

Everybody leaves home in the morning or at birth
For a job, for a purpose or for a cause
Let me do my job well so I can go home
I must go home and everything must go home.

I need to balance my mind and life,
To find freedom, joy, and happiness in life
Then home is near
Home is sweet, home is love, and home is comfort
Home is the rest, home is everything
Let's go home, let's go home!

CHAPTER SIX

Defining Health, Happiness, Disease & Suffering

Everyone wants to be healthy and happy, and there is no question about it. Equally interesting and intriguing is the fact that most people do not know what is meant by health or happiness. For example, if I ask you what is meant by health or happiness, either you will not be able to explain to me in clear language or you will fumble. You may also not be able to explain to me clearly whether or not you are healthy. One of the reasons is that most of the people are neither healthy nor sick; they fall between the two opposite ends of the spectrum—health on one end and disease on the other end. Therefore let us understand and define few terms in this reference, so that we are at the same level of understanding.

I also want you to know that the word health is not properly defined by most of the medical books or even the dictionary. Ayurveda is the only medical science that has given a complete and precise definition of health, and it covers all three aspects of health: physical, mental, and spiritual. Let me summarize the definition of health as given by Ayurveda in few words: "One who has good appetite, whose senses (ear, eye, nose, throat, tongue, and skin) are healthy, whose mind is balanced, and one who is content and blissful, is a healthy person."

The point I am trying to make is that the complete definition of health should cover all three aspects of health: physical, mental, and spiritual. Health is not the mere absence of disease.

Objectives - Understanding

1. What is health and happiness?
2. What is disease and suffering?

Definitions

Disease – dis (not) + ease, or not at ease, or discomfort; an abnormal bodily condition that impairs functioning which can be usually diagnosed with symptoms. Sickness means ill health, also known as nausea.

Suffering – disturbed feeling, agony, anguish, misery, and woe. Remember the word feeling is a subjective rather than an objective phenomenon. For example, if one is diagnosed with heart disease, then suffering will be fear, depression, anger, or guilt as a result of the disease. So a diseased person may or may not be the victim of suffering.

Health – sound, physical, and mental well-being. For complete and perfect definition of health. I shall refer you to Chapter 37: Ayurveda.

Happiness – sound physical or mental health, plus contentment and adeptness; these later components reflect the spiritual health. Therefore happiness is indicative of physical, mental, and spiritual health.

Healing – becoming whole or complete. Healing and curing are similar words, whereas palliation is not becoming whole. It is only the relief of the symptoms.

Health: physical, mental, spiritual differentiation

Since total health has three components, i.e., physical, mental, and spiritual, let me clarify the differences between them in several ways. For example, I could compare these three levels with reference to education, age, or mental growth and/or maturity, and so on.

Education

Physical, mental, and spiritual health in reference to education can be shown as follows: Physical health corresponds to middle school, mental health to college, and spiritual health to post-doctorate.

Age

Physical, mental, and spiritual health in reference to age can be shown as follows: Physical health corresponds to young adults or youth. Mental health usually corresponds to the early part of middle age. Spiritual health corresponds to the mature years of life and/or inner awakening.

We all know young adults who are physically healthy and strong. They may not be mentally as strong because they have not dealt with many challenging situations in life yet.

In the early part of middle age, one gets smarter and more balanced because one has dealt with many challenging situations in life. However, one may not be as strong physically as one was ten or twenty years ago, but one is definitely far more mentally stable.

By the mature years of life, one becomes more adept and content. One has seen many harsh realities of life and has learned that all situations and hardships are part of life and they keep on coming at their own pace. One further learns to appreciate that real peace and comfort lie within the heart and soul. One cannot afford to lose peace over the little issues of life.

Mental growth and maturity

Physical, mental, and spiritual health in reference to mental growth and/or maturity can be demonstrated as follows: In this reference I would like to quote from Prophet Edgar Cayce. "For, we are—physically—what we have digested for the body. We are mentally that which we have thought, but it hasn't added one whit to the physical, has it? We are spiritually that which we have digested in our mental beings."

Now let me summarize and simplify the definition of physical, mental, and spiritual health.

Physical health

The hallmarks of good physical health are physical strength and stability, or the ability to deal with or face the physical challenges of life effectively, such as heat and cold, disease and suffering, injury and pain. One may have the following qualities:

A. Good appetite and digestion
B. Good senses (eyes, ear, nose, tongue, skin)
C. Sound sleep
D. Good physical energy
E. Strong back
F. Strong legs
G. Ideal weight

If you take the example of youth, they may have the following additional qualities:

H. No fear of death
I. Willingness to take chances
J. Willingness to explore

Mental health

The hallmarks of good mental health are mental strength and stability, or the ability to handle stress and meet the new trying situations and challenges with calmness and clarity of mind. They are the result of:

A. Presence of mind
B. Balance of mind
C. Balance of emotions
D. Balance of ego
E. Good intellect

Spiritual health

The hallmarks of good spiritual health are spiritual strength and stability. It has two components.

1. At the personal level: One is adept, content, and satisfied within the self. One appreciates and enjoys life.

2. At the interpersonal level: One has the feeling of oneness, so that one becomes kind and loving to all.

Disease and sub-clinical diseases and states

I have mentioned before that health and disease are at opposite ends of the spectrum. In other words, there must be a big gap between the two. Let us try to understand the sub-clinical diseases and/or states that fill that gap.

There are so many diseases that if I just make a list of them, it will take approximately three to four hundred pages. The typical reference is the I.C.D. book (*International Classification of the Disease*). Now if you take the sub-clinical diseases, there are several times more than the diseases listed in the I.C.D book. Furthermore, that book does not list sub-clinical diseases, nor does it list many mental diseases and none of the spiritual diseases.

Let me give you some examples of diseases that are not listed. I have no complaint as to why they are not listed, because there must be a reason. Probably one of the reasons is that people believe that they are not treatable or curable.

Examples of physical diseases and sub-clinical states

Let us take the example of arthritis, which is a disease. If a person has pain in the knee for five minutes every day, it would not be considered arthritis, because it is in a sub-clinical disease state.

Let us say when a person sits for more than one hour and then gets stiff for ten minutes or so, he will not be labeled as arthritic, but he is suffering from the condition. Similarly when a person complains about joint pain on a rainy day, he would not be labeled as arthritic. So in reference to each disease there are so many sub-clinical states.

Let me give you the example of insomnia, which is a diagnosis. For example, if a person cannot sleep once every three to four weeks, he or she will not be labeled as insomniac. Or if someone wakes up at four o'clock in the morning once a week and cannot go back to sleep, he or she will not be diagnosed as suffering from insomnia. Or if someone takes two hours to fall asleep but then sleeps well, he or she will not be treated for insomnia. The point that I want to make is there are so many sub-clinical states for each conditions and for each disease that one should be aware of.

Let me clarify by giving one more example. A patient comes to me and states that when he took his blood pressure at a pharmacy, it was 140/90. But when I checked in my office, it was 120/80. Now I cannot label him as suffering from high blood pressure. I hope I have made my point clear to you.

Examples of mental diseases and sub-clinical states

Mental diseases include mania, fear, anxieties, and worries. There are many sub-clinical states that do not fall into the above categories. For example, a person gets sad once every two weeks for one day, but he will not be labeled or treated as being depressed. A patient who cannot sleep the night before his flight because of the fear of flying will not be labeled as having an anxiety disorder and will not be treated as such. Somebody who has fear of death or fear of darkness will not be treated or labeled as one with a panic disorder.

Examples of spiritual diseases and sub-clinical states

Spiritual diseases are worse than mental and physical diseases as a cause of pain, suffering, and destruction. Examples of spiritual diseases are: anger, jealousy, greed, habitual stealing, theft, racism, hating someone, being selfish, and being mean.

Of course there are different grades and shades of these diseases, but they are not listed for two possible reasons:

1. The patient is in total denial.
2. It does not fall in the treatment scope of the physician or the psychiatrist.

These are hard to treat. The real treatment comes only from inner awakening, which belongs to only the few and fortunate ones.

What is health?
When appetite is good and belly soft
When head is cool and feet warm
When back is flexible and legs strong
When energy is balanced and one feels strong
It is a sign of physical health

When emotions are in control
When brain is sharp and intellect keen,
When mind is balanced, and one is calm
It is a sign of mental health

When one is content and adept
When one is happy and at peace
When one treats others as brother/sister
It is sign of spiritual health.

The next section is the largest of all the sections in this book. It is devoted to the practical aspects of how to be healthy at the physical, mental, and spiritual levels.

I would like to suggest that if you are clear so far, to feel free to move to the next section. However, if you have any doubt, please review those portions that are unclear to you before proceeding, or just move on.

SECTION II

How to be Healthy & Stay Healthy

I have already devoted one whole chapter to defining health. Now it is the time for us to move on to the practical side of health. I will discuss each and every element of our life at the levels of the body, mind, and soul, and I will demonstrate how to be healthy and strong with little techniques, formulas, and suggestions. I will also do my best to make the information simple, practical, and easy to follow.

This section is divided into three chapters, corresponding to the three levels of our existence.

Let us begin…

CHAPTER SEVEN

Physical Health: Definition

This chapter deals with details on the practical side of physical health. However, it is important not to lose sight of the fact that physical health is part of the physical, mental, and spiritual health trio, and not a separate entity.

Since this subject is so vast and important, let us review the definition of physical health one more time: Physical health can be defined as the strength and stability of the body, and it is directly proportional to good functioning of all the physical organs; for example, good digestion, strong sensory organs, strong heart, lungs, liver, kidneys, back, legs, and so on.

Physical health also equates to the ability to face or deal with all the physical challenges of life effectively; e.g., heat and cold, disease and suffering, injury and pain, and so on.

Physical health in youth

Here are the features/attributes of physical health in youth:

1. They don't get tired.
2. They enjoy a good appetite and good digestion.
3. They get sound and refreshing sleep.
4. They have a beautiful or handsome body.
5. They have no fear, anxiety or worries.
6. They do not fear death.
7. They desire to learn and experiment.
8. They are ready to take chances.

The final result is an abundance of physical energy.

The opposite of physical health

1. They have diseases and sub-clinical diseases.
2. They face diseases at early or younger age.
3. They suffer chronic sickness or get sick from slightest causes.

The result is a lack of energy and stamina, a multiplicity of diseases, and poor health.

CHAPTER EIGHT

Physical Body

In this chapter I discuss the layout of the body. What are its various organ systems? How do these systems function? How can we keep them healthy?

Objective

Understanding the body, its layout, and functioning.

Understanding the body and its layout

It is amazing how beautifully your body is engineered! How beautiful is the architecture! How complete and independent is your body! It can be compared with almost any other system in the world. It shows that everything in the universe is complete in itself, autonomous in nature.

For precise and thorough understanding of the body, let us compare our body with the sugar factory one more time.

I have done this comparison earlier in the chapter "Who Am I." I do not mind repeating it here, because it does serve the purpose well. However, in this chapter I shall expand more on the physical aspect of it.

In order to understand the functioning of the sugar factory, first we need to understand the layout of the factory. This is not very different from our body's systems.

The sugar factory building has three floors. The building itself stands on four pillars and has two extensions. In the factory, on the first floor the raw sugar cane (food) is brought in. It is crushed, juice is prepared, and the pulp or the fiber is thrown out. On the second floor the juice is circulated, heated and purified, and thus converted into sugar. On the third floor are the executive offices of the factory. It has windows and cameras for surveillance and monitoring. The factory has a lobby (mouth) for business dealing.

Now let us compare this sugar factory with our body. The first floor of the sugar factory corresponds to our abdomen. We eat the food, and then it is digested and converted into juices. The stool and urine that are excreted correspond to the pulp or fiber of the sugar cane. The second floor corresponds to our chest. In the chest are the heart and lungs. Here blood is oxygenated and carbon dioxide is eliminated, and then blood is moved into circulation. The third floor of the sugar factory belongs to the executive offices, which correspond to our head and brain. You know our head is equipped with eyes, ear, and nose which are like the surveillance cameras. Our mouth corresponds to the lobby. We use our mouth to meet and greet others. Then there are two poles (two legs) on which our body is standing. (These two poles are so unique that they help the body to walk wherever our mind wants to take the body.

Then we have two arms, which are like extensions of the factory, where all shipping and receiving take place. So our body is like a walking factory.

Nine doors

Our body (building) has nine openings or doors, as follows:

1. Six openings are the sensory organs for the reception of the information from the external world. These are two eyes, two ears, and two nostrils. These are like the little surveillance cameras of a factory.

2. There are two points of exit, the rectum, and the urethra. Here all the waste products are eliminated. These two organs are also known as

organs of excretion. (Stool and urine correspond to the waste pulp of the sugar cane.)

3. The ninth opening is the mouth. The mouth has an important role to play. It can be compared with the main lobby of a factory. You all know the importance of what goes on in a lobby of any organization. Similarly it is important to know what goes into the mouth as food and what comes out of the mouth in the form of words.

The body as one unit with multiple systems

Our physical body consists of several systems that correspond to several departments of a factory. All systems work in coordination with each other for the benefit of the body's systems. All systems have a unique job to perform, but all systems are very much interdependent; so much so that if any system does not function properly, all other systems suffer.

That is also the case with one's body. In it, every system is dependent upon each other for its needs. If any of the organ systems becomes weak or diseased, all other systems suffer to some extent. For example, an upset stomach means less energy production for every system. If one has a breathing problem, all systems take the punch. Similarly if circulation is affected, it has a negative effect on every system. When the brain does not function properly, all systems do not coordinate, as happens in a stroke. If one has a disease of the skin, it is not only a skin disease, but it also reflects malfunctioning of the whole body. It is important to understand that the human body is not two, three or more units, but just one interconnected system.

The functioning of each system

Digestive system

It is the only system that produces physical energy (different from mental, intellectual, or spiritual energy). All other systems are totally dependent for their physical energy needs on the digestive system. In later years of life, one of the causes of weaknesses of all the systems is that they do not get adequate energy from the digestive system. Of course, other systems also get weak with the aging process.

Respiratory system (oxygen, the breath of life)
With each act of breathing, we take in not only oxygen but also energy (*prana*). We also get rid of carbon dioxide with each breath. Most people may not be aware of the fact that we take in energy with each act of breathing. Energy is also known as *chi* or *prana*. Remember each deep breath gives us more energy than a superficial breath. You will learn later how to get more energy from each act of breathing.

Circulatory system
The role of the circulation is to keep the blood flowing or keep the energy in motion. With the flow of blood, each and every tissue, each and every cell in the body gets nourishment (from the final product of digestion and from the act of breathing). Furthermore, each cell and tissue discharges carbon monoxide and waste products into the blood, which is carried back to the kidneys, liver, lungs, and skin for purification and/or excretion.

Excretion system
The four organ systems here are the kidneys, bowels, lungs, and skin. The body wants to get rid of the unnecessary and unwanted chemicals by the kidney and rectum. Carbon dioxide is eliminated by the lungs. The skin finishes the job.

Skeletal system
This system provides protection, support, and/or both. Without the help of the bony support, we would not be able to use our hands so firmly and our legs would not support us in walking or standing. Without our backbone, we would not be able to stand erect. Without this protection, our delicate brain, lungs, and heart would not be able to survive the harsh environment.

Reproductive system
The purpose of the system is the propagation of the human species or to avoid extinction.

Skin
The skin acts like a barrier between the body and the external environment. It also provides a cooling mechanism through perspiration, and also acts as an excretory organ.

Nervous system

Its main role is the coordination of all other systems. In the first step, it receives the information from each and every system, and also from the external world with the help of the eyes, ears, nose, tongue, and skin. Now the brain coordinates all of this information and sends messages back to each and every cell, tissue, and system for its execution.

Endocrine system

This delicate system stands high in the hierarchy of systems. It is responsible for hormone production. It is affected by emotions, feeling, sadness, and happiness. There are seven sets of endocrine glands, including: pituitary, pineal, thyroid, thymus, pancreas, adrenals, and sex glands. The sex glands are testes in males and ovaries in females. The many vital functions of our body are governed by the hormones secreted from these glands.

How to strengthen physical systems for health and well being

In subsequent chapters, we will learn how to strengthen each and every system in our body. This information is practical, simple, and useful. It is neither theoretical nor complex. Every reader can benefit from this information.

Let us start with the digestive system, because all other systems depend on it for their physical energy needs.

CHAPTER NINE

Digestion: Appetite for Food, Appetite for Life

We need energy. Everybody needs energy. Energy is health. We can get energy in many ways, e.g., food, breathing, rest, sleep, exercise, meditation, and so on. But still, food is the commonest and easiest external source of energy.

You must be as amazed as I am as to how milk, bread, cheese, ice cream, grains, beans, vegetables, fruit, and meat become energy. Is it not just short of magical? Food cannot provide energy until it is first digested. So the main role of the digestive system is to convert food into a usable source of energy for the body. It is the only system can do this job.

Remember even the most nutritious and healthiest foods are useless until they are first digested. Every type of food, good or bad, first has to interact with the digestive system, which is like a gatekeeper. It can welcome or reject (vomiting or diarrhea) any food it wishes. The importance is the digestive system can be further understood by the fact that during any sickness, acute or chronic, our digestive system is weak.

A weakened digestive system is probably also the first sign of aging. So it is important to know how our digestive system functions, and what we can do to maintain its good and proper functioning.

Objectives

1. The role of the digestive system is to convert food into energy.

2. The physical health of a person is directly and proportionately related to the good functioning of the digestive system to a great extent.

3. Many diseases, if not all, have their origin in a weak digestion, especially in later years.

4. We can improve and maintain the functioning of the digestive system with a little education and training.

Introduction

We are what we eat, and also we eat what we are. Whatever we eat becomes part of our blood and eventually of our body. Food also has physical, mental, and spiritual energy, just like the blood or the body. Blood is like juice of the ingested food after the digestive process is completed; therefore it is important to choose the food carefully.

Blood may look similar but it is very different in energy. I am not talking about the blood grouping, which is a different subject. You know when you crush mangoes you get mango juice; when you crush oranges you get orange juice. Similarly blood is the juice of the food we eat. Analyze carefully how different people choose different foods. Warriors, soldiers, and fighters prefer hot food and animal food to make them strong physically, even at times at the cost of mental acuity.

On the other hand, intellectual and spiritual people usually prefer simple foods in moderate amounts, which are easier on the stomach and help to maintain good functioning of the brain. They prefer fruits, vegetables, milk, and they may or may not eat fish.

Spiritual people prefer fruits, vegetables, grains, milk and other foods, which not only are digested easily but which also have spiritual energy. Such foods are usually served in temples. Spiritual people usually do not prefer food of animal origin, such as eggs, fish, chicken, or meat, because these foods do not have spiritual energy. It is possible that spiritual energy dies when an animal is killed. Remember the meat that people eat comes from the bodies of dead or killed animals, so think about this carefully before choosing your food.

Definition of digestion

Digestion is defined by the dictionary as follows: breakdown of food in the stomach and intestine into a substance that can be used by the body.

How our digestive system functions

Digestion of food is a complex process. The function of digestion is to convert food into blood. It is not an easy process. Can you imagine how bread, milk, grains, fruits, vegetables, meat, or anything you eat becomes blood? It is a tough job!

The entire alimentary tract, including the stomach, small bowels, colon, liver and pancreas, works in coordination with each other in this process from the time food is eaten to the time blood is formed.

Our body uses as much as 25 to 30 percent of its energy to digest food. Repeated animal experiments show that animals that are fed less live longer and healthier vs. their counterparts. The majority of people in United States eat much more than their needs, therefore they make their digestive system overwork and tire. Overeating is probably one of the most common causes of weak digestion and hence an invitation to diseases.

The digestive system has four components:

1. Ingestion, the process of ingesting the food (eating)

2. Digestion, breaking down the food into smaller particles for conversion into →chyle

3. Assimilation, the incorporation of the digestive element into the body and body tissues

4. Elimination, ridding the body of waste products (stool)

Ingestion

Your body is the product of the food you eat. You should eat food with due and careful consideration. This fact cannot be over-emphasized. You should not eat food out of boredom, fun, sadness, nervousness, or depression. If you wish to have fun foods, you could have them perhaps once a week or at parties. Or the best thing is to learn to enjoy healthy food. Ingestion is the only component of the digestive system over which you have voluntary control.

You have no control of the other three components of the digestive processes, so use all of your intelligence and awareness in deciding what food you should eat. Certainly you should never eat in the absence of appetite. Eating in the absence of appetite is a load that has a significant negative effect on the body.

Digestion

The stomach has to digest whatever you eat. From here on, you have no choice. (Even if you eat poison, the stomach has to digest it.) In the process of digestion, food is broken down into molecules of proteins, fats, and carbohydrates which in turn become part of the chyle→blood. If you eat the right amount and right kind of food, it will digest easily and provide good health. Conversely if you eat the wrong food or an excessive amount of even the right food, you may suffer from indigestion and disease.

Assimilation

In this process all the digestive elements become part of the body's tissue. At first, the digested food becomes chyle, and then it goes through the following schema:

Chyle→to blood→to fat→to muscles→to brain→ to bones→ to nerves→ to semen→etc.

(This schema is taken from Ayurvedic literature.)

You know that certain people, no matter what they eat, cannot gain an ounce of weight or they get diarrhea. This means they have a poor assimilation power and hence cannot incorporate digested food into their body tissues.

Elimination

The whole alimentary tract from the mouth to the anus is one closed system; there are no openings anywhere in between them. Getting rid of the indigestible residue (stool) is known as the process of elimination. When you are constipated or when you can't move bowels without help (laxative, tea, etc.), it means your whole digestive system is weak or below par.

The relationship of digestion to health

Digestion and physical health are very much related. When I was a little child, one of our Swami Ji used to visit us often. He always used to ask us two questions:

1. How much food do you eat in a day?
2. How many times you recite gyatri mantra (mantra to increase the intellect)?

It did not make any sense to me at that time, but now I realize why he used to ask those two questions. The stronger your digestion is, the better your physical health will be. Stronger digestion also has a positive effect on mental sharpness.

You will also observe that the majority of healthy people have good digestion, and conversely most sick people have weak or poor digestion. In almost all acute diseases, patients lose their appetite. Examples of acute diseases are fever, flu, cold, diarrhea, pneumonia, and so on.

In most chronic diseases, patients usually do not have a good appetite or they have decreased the ability to digest food. Thus food causes belching, bloating, acidity, gas, constipation, abdominal pain, and other problems.

It may be hard to establish a cause-and-effect relationship of weak digestion with disease, but these often co-exist. Whenever digestion improves, the health also improves and disease becomes more manageable or it even disappears. So it should be our paramount duty to keep our digestive system strong for better health.

Digestion as a metaphor

The word digestion is used not only for the digestion of the food but also for understanding information at the mental level. For example, when we are teaching a subject that is new and difficult, we often say let's digest this information before we go to the next step.

The common problems of the digestive system

Since I have mentioned that food is the source of all physical energy, let us discuss some of the common problems of the digestive system. In this section I will discuss three problems: constipation, diarrhea, and GERD.

Constipation

Constipation is a serious disease. It is not only a sign of a weakened digestive system, but also an indication of weakened vitality. It is the forerunner of multiple diseases. Many authorities label constipation as a hydra-headed complaint.

Constipation means that one is unable to move bowels at least once a day without the aid of a laxative, tea, or coffee. A healthy bowel movement takes place the first thing in the morning without eating, without tea or coffee, and it comes spontaneously without any aid or pushing.

If you cannot move your bowels spontaneously, think carefully and plan to take some corrective action in the form of exercise, fasting, or change of diet. Try your best not to use laxatives and purgatives, if possible. Remember bowel movements that happen with the help of laxatives or any other aid do not correct the weakness of the digestive system. Rather, chronic use of laxatives has weakening effect on the gastro-intestinal system. The main causes of constipation are too much food, the wrong food (too much meat or sweets or too much acidic food) or food that is hard to digest, such as fried food.

Foods that remove constipation (These may differ slightly from person to person.)

Most fruits and vegetables make the body alkaline and remove constipation. Please also understand that apples have a different effect than applesauce. While apples tend to remove constipation, applesauce tends to cause constipation. Bananas may cause constipation or diarrhea, depending on how your body reacts. Overeating usually causes constipation; however overeating can cause diarrhea, too.

Meat and sweets are the next important causes of constipation. Most grains and legumes lack fiber and therefore can cause constipation.

Adding vegetables to grains and legumes is the practical way of avoiding constipation.

Make your own food list

You should make your own list of the foods that makes you constipated or have diarrhea. Whenever you are constipated, eat foods that help you to move your bowels. When you have diarrhea, eat foods that cause you to be constipated. In this way you can balance your bowel movements.

Whenever you get constipated, it is time to take corrective action. Consider the following:

1. Provide rest to your digestive system. Drink liquids or eat soups for one to three days.

2. Drink an adequate amount of water, unless you are very cold.

3. Take only juices or soup, if you are not hungry.

4. Fast for a day or so; at least miss one, two, or three meals in the sequence.

5. If you cannot do that, then drink only juices. Do not eat any grains, legumes, meats, or sweets until your stomach regains its original function.

6. Sip warm water all day, even just a swallow of water. Do not sip cold water because it slows down the digestive system.

Constipation – Ayurveda perspective

According to Ayurveda, constipation is a serious disease. It indicates sluggishness of the bowels and weakness of the system. If you cannot move your bowels, the gases behind the stool get trapped and start to travel backwards and upwards thereby causing reversal of the normal mechanism. As these gases start to go up, they may affect the liver, spleen, stomach, heart, lungs, throat, sinuses, and even brain in reverse order. You may have heard that people can get headaches from constipation. These people are very sensitive to these gases.

If the constipation continues, the fluid contents of the bowels start to travel backwards in reverse order. Most physicians know that when the bowels get obstructed, people vomit food and even stool.

Diarrhea

Diarrhea can be acute or chronic. Chronic diarrhea is a much more serious condition than constipation, because chronic diarrhea drains the body of its nutrients. However, acute diarrhea can usually be managed as follows:

Acute diarrhea is usually a self-limiting condition. You can usually take care of yourself by providing rest to the digestive system. You must avoid all vegetables, fruits, meats, sweets, milk, coffee, and tea. However, you may eat bananas, applesauce (not apples), rice, and toast. You should avoid drinks that have caffeine such as Coke and Dr. Pepper, but you may drink ginger ale, 7-Up, and Gatorade, because these drinks do not contain caffeine, and yet they provide water and electrolytes. Tap water or bottled water should be avoided during diarrhea, because it lacks electrolytes. During diarrhea the replacement of fluids and electrolytes is very crucial. You must make sure that you do not get dehydrated.

GERD

Symptoms of GERD are acidity, heartburn, belching or bloating, and even regurgitation of food. This disease is usually related to acidity of the stomach. It is usually caused by the excessive or incorrect intake of food. It therefore indicates an overwhelmed and exhausted digestive system.

Treatment of GERD
Avoid constipation. Keep the bowels open. Eat alkaline foods, such as fruits and vegetables. Do not eat two to three hours before you go to bed. Avoid foods that are hard to digest, at least in the evening. Still the single most important advice is to eat only fruits and vegetables until your system returns to normal and symptoms of GERD disappear.

Stomach acid is needed for the digestion of food. Antacids and H2 blockers can cause symptomatic relief of the acidity; however they may affect the digestive process negatively by lowering the acidity in the stomach.

Frequently Asked Questions

Is my digestion good?
The indications of good digestion are good appetite and hunger, ability to digest food, and ability to move bowels spontaneously, i.e., without any purgative assistance.

On the contrary, the signs of poor digestion are lack of appetite and hunger, constipation, feeling of being bloated, heartburn, and inability to digest food. These symptoms are forerunners of many physical diseases.

Also remember that whenever the digestive process is not functioning properly, your energy level goes down and diseases start to attack. Diabetes, cancer, tuberculosis, heart attacks, and cholesterol problems are at least partly related to and/or aggravated by poor digestion.

Take the test: Am I hungry or not?
If the question ever arises whether or not you are hungry, think you are not. You will be right generally. Otherwise this question should not have come to your mind. Just pass on the food; you will not suffer, but you

can penalize yourself by overeating. Under-eating does not kill anyone, unless there is a lack of food for a long period of time.

(On the contrary, if the question comes to your mind whether or not you are thirsty, probably you are.)

How often should I eat?

Demand vs. scheduled feeding

Some advocates say that we should eat only when we are hungry; while others prefer three meals a day, i.e., scheduled feeding. There is some controversy about demand vs. scheduled eating. Both theories have pros and cons, but eating without hunger is a load to the body and bad for the health. You can have a combination of demand plus scheduled feeding which I discuss in Chapter 43.

You should not take breakfast for at least one to two hours after getting up in the morning. I'm not talking about tea, juice or coffee, but rather a full breakfast. The reason is that you must give your body time for the appetite to return, unless you have a big appetite or are a child and/or unless you have no digestion problems.

You should definitely avoid all meals until you move your bowels. If you are hungry but have not moved your bowels, you can have fruit, juices, or tea.

How much should I eat?

Eat just the right amount. Eating too much will cause you to become overweight, and eating too little can make you lose weight. In general, you should eat two-thirds of your capacity at any given meal. If your weight is normal and maintained, then you are getting adequate food.

There is an interesting story about Lord Krishna who ate one grain of rice and felt satisfied. This story is depicted in one of the "the greatest epics of India" titled *Mahabharata*. Lord Krishna was one of the greatest souls born in India. Some people call him Bhagwan (Godly Soul).

Here is an authentic story of a lady who never ate food. Swami Parmahansa Yogananda narrates this unique and authentic story in his book titled *Autobiography of a Yogi*. Swami Ji personally visited her and interviewed her.

She told Swami Ji, "I was once criticized that I eat too much; thereafter I decided not to eat. It is my decision," she said. "You can do anything, once you make up your mind." But she refuses to divulge the secret. She stated that if she tells the secret, it will hurt all of the farmers.

How much time does one need to spend eating?
It will vary depending on the amount of food you eat. However, the general principle is that you must chew the food until it becomes liquid. Respect the proverb "Drink your solids and eat your liquids."

Food combinations
Mixing or combining foods is also science and art. Certain groups of foods do not mix well with each other; whereas other groups do mix well. For example, vegetables mix with any food or combination thereof. Fruits do not mix with anything except milk. Two animal proteins do not mix well in any given meal. For example, you should not eat cheese and burger in the same meal. You may either eat either cheese or burger, not together. You may take either fish or milk, not both. You may not eat eggs and bacon together. Ask your Jewish friends; they know that principle very well. They differentiate kosher from non-kosher food. Avoid eating meat with carbohydrates. Eating meat with potatoes or meat with gravy is very hard for digestion.

How much water should we drink?

This is a commonly asked question. Should one drink six to eight glasses a day? I think it is not proper to say that everybody should drink six to eight glasses a day. It depends on the weather conditions, body size, age, activities, foods eaten, and from what disease one has been suffering.

Certainly you should drink enough water, and drink a half hour before each meal and first thing in the morning. Drinking excessive amounts of water can be as bad as not drinking an adequate amount.

If your urine is always yellow, that probably means you are not drinking enough, but if your urine is always clear like water, that means you are drinking enough or too much. This is probably a good guide.

According to the philosophy of Taoism, drinking excessive amounts of water may cause kidney weakness. This point needs some due consideration. Probably most of you know that water pills (to get rid of water) are the #1 drugs used in the treatment of high blood pressure. Therefore you need to understand that drinking excessive water can also be harmful. I do not mean to say that you should not drink adequate water, but what I am saying is that drinking too much water can also cause problems. However, in general, people are relatively dehydrated and drink less water than they should.

Colonics

Colonics do not make any sense to me. You should know that our gut is twenty-eight feet long. The whole gut has food in it in all stages, from freshly eaten food to the last stages (stool). Fresh food lies in the stomach; the stool lies in the rectum; and rest of the gut has food in all different stages. With colonics you are cleaning only the last four to five feet of your colon; you are not cleaning the whole gut. After colonics, the colon is filled again with stool within couple of hours. Also with colonics, you push up germs of the lower colon into the higher colon, which is against the law of nature. According to natural health, the flow in the colon should be from above to below, not below to above.

Sleep before or after meal?

Make sure you do not sleep immediately after eating. On the contrary, taking a ten- to fifteen-minute rest before eating is the good, especially if your digestive process is slow. Taking a nap or siesta after a heavy meal contributes to acidity and gas, and slows down digestion. Resting (not sleeping) ten to fifteen minutes after a meal is okay. You may go to sleep two hours after a meal.

Avoid choking while eating

Choking from food can be avoided by:

1. eating slowly
2. avoiding any conversation while eating
3. leaning forward while eating

Leaning forward allows easy access of food from mouth into the stomach without entering the windpipe. In India, China, and some other eastern cultures, many people sit on the floor to eat. It has one unique advantage: one has to lean forward to ingest foods that prevents choking.

Appetite: a million dollar question

All this information will be incomplete, if I do not discuss the appetite and its importance. It is further interesting to note that this subject is not discussed by practitioners of conventional medicine, nutritionists, and even natural hygienists.

It is extremely important to choose not only the right quality but also the right quantity of food. This can be easily accomplished by understanding your appetite level before each meal and then planning to eat accordingly. In the absence of appetite, even the best selected foods can cause serious problems.

I see dietitians prescribing diets to diabetic patients based on their height and weight. They do not consider how much food one normally eats. For example, if a patient is prescribed a 2,000-calorie diet, and they are used to only 1,500 calories, 500 calories would be a load to this person which can cause further aggravation of their diabetic condition.

Appetite: improve, maintain, and preserve

One of the best secrets to preserve, maintain and improve the appetite is to eat in proportion to the appetite. It is a three point formula

1. Know your level of appetite at every meal. Appetite can be classified as poor, fair, good, or very good.

2. Food can also be classified based upon their digestibility e.g.

    a. Very easy to digest food: fruits and juices

    b. Easy to digest food: yogurt, bread, rice

    c. Little harder to digest foods: balanced meal of grain, beans, vegetables, fruits, nuts, milk, etc.

    d. Very hard to digest foods: everything that I have said so far, plus meat and dessert (In other words, meat and dessert are hard to digest.)

3. Now match the appetite with the digestibility of the food e.g.

    - In the absence of appetite, you can have fruit or fruit juices only. (List a)

    - For fair appetite, you can have fruits and yogurt or toast and rice. (List b)

    - For a good appetite, you can have a balanced meal of grain, beans, vegetables, fruits, and dairy. (List c)

    - If you have a very good appetite, then you can have anything, even animal products, if you so wish.(List d)

Many gastrointestinal problems arise because people do not eat in proportion to their appetite. In general, eating lighter is much better than eating heavy; so one needs to pay attention not only to the quality of food but also the quantity of food.

How to improve and maintain the digestive system for better health (Ayurvedic perspective)

1. Eat only when hungry.

2. Eat only after you have moved your bowels. Many people say they cannot move their bowels until they have their breakfast; this is not good. If that is your problem, just have a cup of tea or juice, or go on a fruit diet for one to three days until your digestive system returns to its normal functioning level.

3. Eat more alkaline foods, i.e., fruits and vegetables. Avoid an excess of acidic foods, especially animal protein (meat, chicken, egg, fish), sweets, and sodas.

4. Don't eat two hours before you go to bed.

5. Don't eat at least one hour after you get up, unless you are very young or hungry.

6. Fast once a week. If you cannot fast or you are underweight, eat only fruits on that day.

7. Never eat to satiety. It is like filling the pot with rice to the brim and then starts cooking.

8. Do not go for second helpings. When you go for seconds, usually you are overeating.

9. Don't eat foods too hot or too cold, both are hard on the stomach. Warm foods are preferable.

10. Don't hesitate to experiment; you must know your body well.

11. Avoid multiple classifications of the foods at any given meal especially if your digestive system is weak. Also do not eat more

than one protein in any given meal, e.g., cheese and burger, fish and milk, eggs and bacon.

12. Avoid meat with carbohydrates (meat with gravy, meat with bread, meat with potatoes). Eat meat with vegetables.

13. Learn to experience and tolerate hunger. When you tolerate hunger, the gut becomes stronger and cleans out the built-in toxins. Also it is an experience just short of fasting.

14. Eat slowly and chew food well until it becomes liquid in mouth.

15. Try to match the qualities and quantities of the food with the degree of your appetite.

Remember the common proverb: Eat breakfast like a king, lunch like a prince, and supper like pauper. Or eat breakfast like a prince, lunch like a king and supper like a pauper.

The key message

Good digestion can provide long life and good health. One can easily learn to maintain good functioning of the digestive system if one is careful enough in choosing:

- The right amount of food
- The right kind of food
- Eating in the right manner
- Eating at the right time
- Most importantly eating in proportion to his or her appetite.

Remember:

When food is good,
And the amount correct,
When appetite is your guide,
And you eat at the correct time,
Then food will give you good health.

CHAPTER TEN

Respiration: The Breath of Life

Respiration is not only one of the most vital functions of life, but also one of the best sources of energy without any cost. The first breath marks the beginning of life, and the last breath terminates life. In this chapter, I will discuss the functions of respiration, the proper breathing technique, and multiple benefits connected to it. I have also included a practical exercise.

No matter how strange it may sound the fact remains the majority of people do not breathe properly. You should know that by breathing properly, you can have more energy, be more clear-headed, be calmer and more relaxed, prolong life, and hence live longer.

Objectives

1. Respiration is the number one necessity for sustenance of life.
2. To learn the art of breathing that provides more energy and better memory, and prolongs life

Introduction

One way to check if a person is alive or dead is to check for two things:

1. Is the person breathing?
2. Does the person have a pulse or is his/her heart functioning?

Definition

The act or process of breathing in (inhaling) and breathing out (exhaling) is known as respiration. Without respiration one cannot live more than three or four minutes, at the most. However, there are authentic stories of yogis who have lived up to forty-five days without breathing. These yogis were buried deep underground for that duration.

The functions of breathing

- During the act of breathing in (inhaling):

1. We intake oxygen from the air.
2. We intake energy, *prana* or *chi,* in addition to oxygen.

- During the act of breathing out (exhaling):

1. We exhale carbon dioxide. (excretion)
2. We also learn to relax with each deep act of exhalation.

- Excretory organ: the respiratory system also acts as one of the four excretory organs of the body. Skin, kidneys, and bowels are the other three. Each of these organs is complementary to the other in the function of excretion. If one of the excretory organs becomes weak, the other three systems have to work harder to compensate.

Breathing as metaphors

The word breathing can be used in a physical and metaphysical sense. When you get bombarded with work, you often say, please let me breathe. It means you need a rest or a break. When you take on a project with firm commitment, you often state, I will not breathe until I finish this project.

We need to appreciate how each word has a physical and metaphysical meaning, just like many things in life.

Breathe better, conserve breaths

It is believed that the number of breaths for one's life is fixed at the time of birth. Maybe it is that after so many breaths, the lungs wear out. The faster you use your breaths, the shorter your lifespan will be. Conversely if you breathe slowly and deeply, you will use fewer breaths and your lifespan will be prolonged.

During any disease or condition when you breathe fast, your lifespan is shortened; this happens in obesity, emphysema, heart failure, and other conditions. Anger, hate, arguments, and rushing also increase the breathing rate and hence shorten the lifespan. Whenever you are doing something bad, you breathe faster. Interestingly whenever you do something good, you are more relaxed and take fewer breaths.

Conserve breaths and live longer

In order to do that, first you must understand how many breaths you take in a minute, in a day, in a year, and in life. Let's say you take 12 breaths per minute. In one hour you will take 720 breaths. In a day you will take 17,280 breaths, and in one year 6,307,200 or 6.3 million breaths. Just imagine if you can cut down the rate of respiration even by one per minute by yogic breathing; that is from 12 to 11 breaths, you will be saving a total of half a million breaths per year! That is quite a saving of breaths. This will result in the prolongation of your life.

The formula to figure out how many breaths you have used in your life is as follows:

Total number of breaths used in life = 6.3 million breaths x age in years. For example, let's say you are 30 years old. Now 6.3 million breaths x 30 equal 189 million breaths. The importance of this equation is to make you conscious of your breathing, so that you breathe properly, that is, slowly and deeply, and you do not waste breaths unnecessarily.

Yogic breathing: Explanation

The yogic breathing technique involves breathing slowly and deeply. This is an ideal way of breathing. There are three components to it:

1. Breathing deeply: as deeply as possible
2. Breathing slowly: as slowly as possible
3. Using abdominal muscles during the act of breathing for full expansion of lungs

During inhalation (breathing in), the abdomen should bulge out like a balloon. During exhalation (breathing out) the abdomen should sink in, and one should try to touch the abdominal muscles to the back. Please be clear about that.

When I try to teach my patients to breathe deeply, some get confused. The common mistake is that they forget that during the act of breathing in, the belly should be ballooning out, because you are taking in air. Spend a few minutes and try to understand this concept. It is worth the time and experience.

If you have a hard time coordinating the act of breathing, lie down on the floor to practice this art, at least in the initial stages. It will be much easier to practice this way. But after you have learned this art of breathing, you should do this exercise while sitting. This is how you should breathe twenty-four hours a day, seven days a week. This is not a mere exercise.

Deep breathing has another advantage. When you breathe deeply and slowly, you use your lungs to their maximum capacity; however when you take shallow breaths, you may use as little as 50 percent of your lungs' capacity.

Deep breathing also results in the stimulation of the parasympathetic nervous system which makes our mind calm. Each inhalation or act of breathing in is an active process for which our body has to function hard, but the process of exhalation is an easy and passive process.

Benefits of yogic breathing, a summary

1. Your mind gets more *prana* or energy.

2. Your mind becomes calm, due to the stimulation of the parasympathetic nervous system.

3. Your mind becomes clearer and more focused.

4. Your memory improves, as more oxygen goes to the brain.

5. Your life gets prolonged (using fewer breaths).

Remember mind and breathing are very much connected to each other. You will notice that people who breathe deeply and slowly are more relaxed.

Yogic breathing exercise

Let us practice the art of yogic breathing to prolong life. Sit down. Be comfortable and relax. Turn off the TV, the phone, and if possible the lights. It is good to be with a group of people who are doing the same practice as you (only if possible).

1. Count the number of breaths you take in one minute. Time it with a watch.

2. Close your eyes. Relax and watch your breaths coming in and going out, from the nostrils for one to two minutes.

3. Start to breathe slowly and deeply. Then more slowly and more deeply. Then a little more slower and little more deeper and so on.

4. Continue this exercise for at least 10 to 15 minutes.

5. Use abdominal muscles during the act of deep breathing.

6. Count again the number of breaths per minute. You will notice that even with this little exercise you will be breathing slower and your body will require fewer breaths per minute. Even if you could save one breath per minute in this practice and maintain that, you will be saving as much as half a million breaths in one year. This should equate to approximately one month added to your life per year of yogic breathing.

Practical Application

1. Prolong life: Conserve the number of the breaths in your life. Practice deep and slow breathing. Don't waste your breath on unnecessary activities. At the physical level: Don't be overweight. Don't smoke. Exercise regularly. At the mental level: avoid anger, arguments, telling lies, and unnecessary rushing.

2. Breathe in (Inhale) consciously to increase *prana* (energy). You can breathe in the energy into your brain, spinal cord, eyes, ear, heart, lungs, and stomach or into any organ to strengthen it.

3. Breathe out (Exhale) consciously to release tension and relax.

4. Use deep breathing for mental relaxation.

5. Increase your energy instantaneously. If you are sitting down and have difficulty getting up, take a long deep breath and hold it. Now try to get up and you will find it much easier to do.

6. If you feel nervous, anxious, and stressed out, close your eyes and start to breathe slowly for three minutes. You will notice it has a calming effect on your body and mind.

CHAPTER ELEVEN

Circulation: On the Go

Circulation and respiration are the two top vital functions of life. Circulation equates to life, and absence of circulation means death. Conversely good circulation means good health, and poor circulation/stagnation/congestion means poor health. We also know how vital the circulation is, especially for the brain. Brain cells begin to die after three to four minutes, if there is no oxygen or circulation to the brain.

Circulation is a universal phenomenon and is not confined to the issue of health. For example, air must be kept in circulation. Money must be kept in circulation. Goods must be kept in circulation. People also move from one place to another whenever the economy is good.

In this chapter we will study the circulatory system, how to improve circulation, and how to live longer by prolonging the life of the heart.

Objectives

1. Circulation is essential for sustenance of life (absence of circulation means death).

2. By improving and normalizing circulation, we can improve the functioning of every system of our body.

3. By improving circulation, we can also slow down the heart rate and prolong life.

Remember everything in the body needs to be kept in circulation: blood, fluid, air, saliva, urine, and so on. When circulation slows down, disease sets in, and when the circulation stops, death occurs.

Circulation: an overview:

Our circulatory system consists of three elements:

1. Heart (pump)
2. Blood vessels (arteries and veins)
3. Blood (fluid)

The heart

The heart is basically a pump. The sole purpose of the heart is to keep the blood pumping. The heart has four chambers (valves). These built-in valves ensure that the blood flows only in one direction. The heart is so important because it is the only organ that cannot rest from the time you are born until the time you die.

Can you imagine the value of an organ that never stops working? (What about the value of people in the family, community, and nation who work non-stop? They are the heart of society.)

You cannot imagine another organ that is more vital than the heart. The average weight of a female human heart is 9 ounces, and a male human heart is 10.5 ounces. The size of the heart is approximately the size of your fist.

Blood vessels (arteries & veins)

The circulatory system is like the transportation system in our community. Transportation systems move things and people from one place to another. Similarly in our body, circulation moves the necessities of life, such as oxygen, carbon dioxide, nutrients, and waste products to their proper destination. The circulatory system is a closed system consisting of the heart, blood, and the blood vessels, including arteries and veins. It is a closed system in the sense that the blood never leaves the blood vessels. (Just like the alimentary tract is a closed system from mouth to anus or rectum, without any openings anywhere.) When the blood reaches the cells and tissues, it liberates oxygen and nutrients and, on its way, removes the carbon dioxide and waste products.

Blood

The blood is the final product of digestion. Whether your blood is healthy and strong or sickly and weak depends greatly upon on the type of food you eat. Blood has two basic components:

1. Cells (red, white, and platelets)
2. Fluid (plasma)

All cells float in plasma, the richest source of protein. Different types of cells perform different functions. Red blood cells carry oxygen from the lungs to the tissues and bring back carbon dioxide. White blood cells fight infection. Platelets are responsible for clotting.

Everything in the body, including the blood, is renewed on a periodic basis. In other words, every day a certain portion of your blood dies and is replaced by an equal amount of new blood. (See Chapter 1) Therefore no matter what your age is, your red blood cells are never more than 120 days old.

The heart as metaphors

I'd like to discuss the following three phrases in this reference:

1. Heart and emotions
2. Heart and soul
3. Big heart

Heart and emotions

The heart and emotions are directly related. The heart is the seat of emotion. When I say "I love you from my heart," it means I love you very much (expression of emotions). When people say "this person has no heart," it does not mean that the person is without a physical heart, but it means they lack feeling. (If somebody could live without a heart, all medical science would fail.) Do not give your heart to anyone; you may need it some day. (Joking) To stay young, you must feel young at heart.

Heart and soul

Remember the heart also has a physical relationship with the soul. According to some yogis, the soul is located in the A.V. node of the heart, although other yogis believe that the seat of the soul is in the pineal gland. Some authorities believe that the soul resides in the medulla oblongata; still other authorities believe that the seat of the soul is in the area between the heart and above.

Big heart

When we say one has a big heart, its interpretation will vary greatly depending in which context it is stated. When we imply that their physical heart is big, it means their heart is enlarged, a diseased condition. But when we imply spiritually, it means they have the quality of a great person. They are broad and open-minded, which is a good quality.

When we want to give encouragement to somebody, we say, "You can do anything if you put your heart and soul in it." Here heart and soul implies one's will and determination. Please remember that the word heart (like many other words) can have a physical, an intellectual, or a spiritual meaning.

How to improve and normalize circulation

There are at least three ways to improve the circulation. There are some other methods also, but the following are easier for an average person to understand:

1. Exercise
2. Massage
3. Tensing and relaxing

Exercise has an important role to play. It not only improves the circulation but also conditions the heart and the body. There are exercises for all levels: physical, mental, and spiritual. (See Chapter 24)

Massage is the second element that can improve circulation. It is good for diseased body parts, for disabled people, and people who are passive. Massage, like any other exercises, should also be done on a regular basis. Ayurveda advocates that it should be done at least once a day.

Tensing and relaxing of body parts will also improve and normalize the circulation and cause one to relax. This is one of the yoga techniques. It is good for people who are confined to a bed or chair.

By improving and normalizing the body's circulation, we can improve not only the functioning of each system but also we can keep the body healthy, clean, and free of toxins.

Live longer: Extend the life of the heart

Life expectancy is directly proportional to the life of the heart. And the life of the heart is directly proportional to its ability to continue to beat. Yogis know that the heart can beat only a certain number of times in one's life. It is as if, after a certain number of beats, the heart wears out, just as the lungs wear out after a certain number of breaths. You can prolong your life by slowing down the heart rate.

Now let's calculate how many times your heart will beat in one year. Let us presume the heart beats at 70 times per minute. In one hour it would beat 4,200 times (70 beats x 60 minutes). In a day it beats 100,800 times (4,200 beats x 24 hours). Or you can round it off to 100,000 times in a day. In a year it will beat 36.5 million times (100,000 x 365 days).

By conditioning or yoga exercises, you can reduce the heart rate from 70 to 60 beats per minute. That is just ten beats per minute. In an hour that means you would conserve 600 beats, and in a day 144,000 beats. In a year you would save 5.2 million beats. You can gain a year of additional life for every seven years of the yoga exercises and conditioning.

Other factors that can prolong life

Physical

- Use energy in positive and useful ways. Do not waste energy on unnecessary activities.

- Eat plenty of vegetables; these are rich in potassium, magnesium, and calcium. Vegetables are also low in cholesterol, fat, and salt. A balanced vegetarian diet has a positive effect on the life of the heart.

- Maintain proper weight. Do not be overweight.

- Exercise for proper conditioning of the heart (decreasing heart rate and increasing endurance).

Mental

- Take your time. Don't rush unnecessarily. There are many situations in life that are not worth stressing over or rushing to do.

- Learn to stay calm and avoid anger. Anger raises one's blood pressure and pulse rate. All wrongful acts also increase the heart rate.
- Enjoy life and relax.

Spiritual

- Observe silence.
- Meditate (to decrease the heart rate and strengthen the heart).
- Learn yogic breathing to improve circulation. (See Chapter 10)

The idea of this book is that if you are determined, not only can you live longer, healthier and happier, but you can also have better control of your life. **This fact cannot be overemphasized**.

So far we have discussed physical health, digestion, respiration, and circulation. In the next chapter we will look at the skeletal system that provides protection and support to our body and its organs.

CHAPTER TWELVE

Skeletal System: Protection & Support

Our bodies have very delicate organs and hence they need to be protected. Our skeletal system serves that purpose very well. In addition, our skeletal system provides firmness and strength to the delicate organs, such as the hands and back. In this chapter we will learn how to keep our skeletal system healthy, strong, and flexible.

Objective

Understanding how to keep our skeletal system healthy, strong, and flexible

Introduction

There are approximately 200 bones in our body. Bones are hard structures.

Function of the skeletal system

The purposes of the bony system are mainly two:

1. Protection
2. Support and strength

The delicate parts of our bodies are protected by bony structures. For example, the brain is protected by the skull; the spinal cord by the spinal column or backbone; and the heart and lungs by the rib cage.

The bony structure also provides firmness, strength, and support to the soft tissues of the body. Without a bony structure, we would not be able to stand on two legs or extend our hands beyond our body.

Medical science deals with bones and joints

There are three types of doctors who deal with the bones and joints: chiropractors, osteopaths, and orthopedic surgeons. Chiropractors deal with the alignment of the back. They believe in manipulation of the back for better health. Osteopaths treat medical disorders through manipulation and massage of the skeleton and musculature. Orthopedic surgeons are medical doctors most highly trained to care for and/or perform surgery on the bones and joints of the body.

How to keep our skeletal system healthy and flexible

Although maintaining general good health will also keep our skeletal system healthy and strong, there are certain specific measures that could provide extra bonuses:

1. Maintaining regular exercise programs for endurance
2. Practicing yoga exercises for the flexibility of the back and body.

The importance of the back for better health cannot be overemphasized. The back serves not only as the supporting structure of the body, but it also protects the nerves and nervous tissue, including the spinal cord. There is no substitute for a well organized yogic exercise program for the back.

3. Keeping the body alkaline: An alkaline body has positive calcium balance and tends to conserve calcium, whereas an acidic body has negative calcium balance and tends to lose calcium. Therefore, one should:

- Eat alkaline food, at least five servings of fruits and vegetables per day. Vegetables are more important than fruits because of their relatively richer source of proteins and calcium.

- Avoid excessive amounts of acidic foods, such as meat, sodas, sweets, tea, and coffee. Acidic foods cause negative calcium balance.

4. Limited exposure to the sun. The sun's rays strengthen the bony structure by providing vitamin D. However excessive sun exposure can cause skin cancer. According to the old textbooks, it is best to avoid direct sun ray exposure from 10 a.m. to 2 p.m. in winter and 10 a.m. to 3 p.m. in summer. Also you should limit the exposure to the sun to a brief period of time.

Exercise: Strengthen your legs in one minute per day

Do this yogic exercise to improve circulation and nerve flow, and to strengthen the legs. This is one of the common yogic exercises that should be done on regular basis:

- Lie on the floor on your back. Relax for thirty seconds.

- Lift the legs into the air **without support** at a 30-degree angle.

- Hold them for one minute in the air. In the beginning one may have difficulty, but with practice one should be able to accomplish this.

- Do this exercise in the morning and in the evening.

Osteoporosis

This is a disease of aging bones that affects some individuals more than others. However everyone is affected to some degree in old age. The health of the bones can be improved to a great extent by following the guidelines given in this section. The use of vitamin D is also encouraged. You should consult your physician for personal care.

CHAPTER THIRTEEN

Skin: Reflection of Health

Our skin reflects our inner health. It is not merely an external covering. Healthy skin is an indication of a healthy body, and diseased skin indicates a diseased body.

Objectives

1. The condition of your skin corresponds with the condition of your general health.

2. The only way to improve the look and feel of the skin is by improving your general health. This fact cannot be overemphasized.

Introduction

If you analyze carefully the skin of an infant, of a child, of a young man, an old man, an athlete, or a sick person, each is different and gives a different impression. Similarly the skin of a yogi or spiritual man gives a different impression. When you look at fruit, vegetables, a piece of cloth, or a kernel or a grain, you can usually tell if it is real or fake, fresh or stale, young or old, ripe or unripe, good or bad, and so on. Such is the importance of the look and appearance of the skin.

Your skin also protects your body from the external environment, from the sun, heat, inclement weather, bacteria, insects, and so on. It is the first organ to come in contact whenever two people meet in an act of love or war.

Your skin is always young. It is constantly renewed and is never more than a few months old, no matter how old a person may be. If you recall that in Chapter 1 on the dynamics of health, we learned how every tissue is replaced by newer and younger tissue at regular intervals. However the new skin that is laid down is similar to the old skin; that is why it does not look any younger. In order to analyze the skin properly, you should look at its color, texture, elasticity, shine, clarity, and so on.

Definition

According to the dictionary, skin is the outer limiting layer of the body. It is made of tougher tissue like any other external covering. Skin also means hide.

Skin as a metaphor

Do you know what it means when people say "save your skin"?

Skin size and area

The area of the skin of the four extremities in an adult is slightly greater than 50 percent of the body skin area. The torso and the head constitute the remaining 50 percent. The area of the head alone is approximately 9 percent.

In cold weather, it pays to cover your extremities and head to prevent heat lost. And in hot weather you should also cover your head to avoid undue exposure from the sun.

Growth and repair

Your skin is always young and new. That is the dynamics of the skin. If you remember at the time of birth, you had a very small skin area. As you grew in size, the newly laid skin also became larger to keep pace with the growing body. When your body shrinks, whether due to old age or weight loss, your newly laid skin also gets smaller in size to keep up with the new demands.

Functions of the skin

The skin has at least three important functions to perform:

- Protection
- Excretion
- Perspiration (a cooling mechanism)

Protection

The skin protects us from the external environment. It separates our body from the outer world.

Organ of excretion

The skin is one of the four organs of excretion. The others are the lungs, kidneys, and bowels. When any of the excretory organs loses it functions or does not function adequately, the skin has to work harder to make up for the deficiency. For example, if you are suffering from kidney, lung or bowel disease, your skin will be unhealthy because of built-in toxins.

Perspiration: a cooling mechanism

Whenever your body gets hot, either due to excessive heat, fever or from exercise, your skin perspires to cools off your body.

Practical Applications

Skin: make it look good and healthy

General health

Anything that improves the general health will also improve the health of the skin, such as healthy diet, exercise, massage, and a happy life.

Massage

Ayurveda recommends that we massage our skin (body) with oil every day. This improves the circulation, get rids of the dead skin more easily, and also it gives a newer and younger look. Everybody can learn how to do a self-body massage.

Local treatment

Treating the skin with lotions and creams has only a temporary effect, because the skin that you have today will be replaced by new underlying skin within months.

Pores

Many people are concerned with skin pores. They try to close them for the sake of vanity, but this can be quite harmful. The pores have a purpose; they eliminate toxins from the body. Antiperspirants close the pores. Beautiful and healthy skin does not need any makeup.

Perspiration

Perspiration is a valuable function that improves the condition of the skin, eliminates toxins, and improves general health; therefore you should perspire as often as possible.

Remember that a healthy fresh-looking skin indicates a healthy body; conversely a diseased looking skin indicates an unhealthy body.

CHAPTER FOURTEEN

Reproductive System: Continuation of the Human Race

Every child brings a message to the world that God is not disgusted with mankind as yet (source unknown).

Every living being wants to live forever. However, that is not possible. Reproduction is the second choice.

Objectives

1. Reproduction is a function of good physical and mental health.
2. The real way to improve the functioning of the reproduction system is to improve the general health.

Introduction and duty

A healthy body means a healthy reproductive system, a good sex life, and healthy children.

We all know that reproduction is essential for continuation of the species. Therefore it becomes our duty to the world to produce only strong and healthy children for the continuation of a healthy human race.

Understanding the value of semen

Semen is a precious element, according to Ayurveda and Taoism. The amount of semen produced is directly proportional to the amount of food eaten, digested, and assimilated. However, the conventional medical world does not give due importance to semen.

Maharishi Swami Dayanand Saraswati (a Vedic scholar) has stated that sex should be used for reproduction only. He stresses the fact that we should strive for mental and spiritual pleasures that are far superior to the physical pleasures of life.

Taoism recommends sex without ejaculation. Doctor Stephen T. Chang in his book *The Tao of Sexology* (the book of infinite wisdom) has given a beautiful description of how to control ejaculation. He calls it a million-dollar point. It is also important to note that those people who lose their semen excessively (especially in later years) suffer from poor health.

Practical points

The real way to improve the functioning of the reproductive system is by improving your physical and mental health. You can do so by choosing healthy food, exercising regularly, and getting adequate rest. At the mental level, you need to stay positive, strong, and balanced.

Semen is a life-giving fluid and not a mere discharge; therefore you should conserve semen at least in later years of life for a better health. You can have sex without ejaculation. Read *The Tao of Sexology* by Dr. Stephen Chang.

Every parent has a duty, an obligation, to produce only strong and healthy children or else future generations will be in trouble. Are you with me on this issue?

In the next chapter we will discuss a very important system that has the responsibility of coordinating all of the systems of the body. This is the central nervous system.

CHAPTER FIFTEEN

The Central Nervous System: Our Command Center

Your nervous system is like the command center or control tower. It controls each and every structure and function of your body.

Objectives

1. The nervous system plays the role of a command center.

2. By improving the functioning of the central nervous system we can also improve the functioning of all other systems.

Understanding the nervous system

Introduction

The nervous system consists of the brain, spinal cord, and nerves. The brain is located in the top of the head. Probably this is the best location, because from there it is easy to monitor the external environment with the help of the eyes, ear, and nose. It is the only system that coordinates all of the activities of the body, voluntary and involuntary.

Nerves as a metaphor

When people say, "I have bad nerves," they are speaking metaphorically. They are saying they have a mental instability or are affected by emotions much more than other people.

Definitions

The nervous system is a bodily system that in vertebrates is made up of the brain and spinal cord, nerves, ganglia, and parts of the sensory organs. It receives and interprets stimuli and transmits nerve impulses. It is important to differentiate the brain from the mind.

The brain, is an organ located in the head, controls the body's functions. The brain is a physical organ that one can touch, see, and feel; whereas the mind is a very subtle element that no one can see or touch in the physical sense. These two words—mind and brain—are not interchangeable in any sense. You can say the brain is a hardware and the mind is the software.

I have devoted one full chapter to the mind, which is a higher element with a dominating and controlling effect on the brain and all systems of the body.

Structure and divisions

Our nervous system consists of two divisions: voluntary and involuntary. The voluntary system is also known as somatic nervous system. It controls all of those activities of life that are under the voluntary control of the mind.

The involuntary nervous system controls those activities in which the decision of the brain is not required. These are vital processes of the body, such as digestion, breathing, circulation, defense, healing, and so on. The involuntary nervous system is also known as autonomic nervous system.

The nervous system: How does it function?

Each and every tissue or cell of the body is connected to the brain with the help of nerves, ganglia, and plexus. In the first step, the brain receives messages from each and every organ or system. It also receives the information from the external world with the help of the eyes, ears, nose, tongue, and skin. The nerves that bring messages to the brain have a special name and are known as *afferent nerves*.

Your brain analyzes and interprets all information. After analysis, it sends back messages or feedback to each and every organ by another set of nerves, known as *efferent nerves*. This is how the nervous system not only governs all other systems but also provides coordination for the other systems. Without the proper functioning of the brain, you would become a vegetable.

The functions of the nervous system

1. The somatic nervous system coordinates each and every voluntary activity of the body.

2. Nerves have a nourishing element. Whenever any part loses its nerve supply, it may end up in atrophy.

3. The autonomic nervous system plays an active role in controlling the vital functions of the body. These are the functions where the brain does not have to think and analyze, for example, breathing, digestion, sleep, and so on. These are done automatically. The automatic nervous system also has two components:

    a. The sympathetic nervous system keeps one alert and prepares one for stressful situations, such as a fight or flight phenomenon. People who easily get nervous and agitated have the "A" personality and have an overactive sympathetic nervous system.

    b. The parasympathetic nervous system makes us relax, calm, and peaceful. This component has a charging and energizing effect on the brain, body, and mind. People who do yoga regularly have a much stronger and more balanced nervous system than those who do not. Yoga not only calms down the sympathetic nervous system, but also strengthens the parasympathetic nervous system.

4. Vigilance. Our brain receives information from the external world with the help of eyes, ears, nose, tongue, and skin and then uses the information for the benefit and protection of the body.

Practical Application

Strengthen the nervous system for better health

It should be clear by now that by improving the functioning of the nervous system, you can also improve the functioning of all other systems. The functioning of the nervous system can be improved in several ways:

1. Healthy nourishment
2. Relaxing the mind, playing, hobbies, creative work
3. Neuro-linguistic programming
4. Meditation.(a spiritual component of yoga)
5. Yoga - With the help of yoga, you can (a) calm down the sympathetic nervous system, (b) stimulate the parasympathetic nervous system, and (c) develop control of the involuntary functions of the body.
6. Observing silence
7. Self-hypnosis

CHAPTER SIXTEEN

The Endocrine Gland System: System of Hormones

The endocrine gland system is the subtlest of all physical systems of the body. It forms a link between the body and the mind or psyche (the metaphysical element). The effects of the endocrine glands on the body are profound. They affect each and every cell, tissue, and nerve. These glands are easily affected by feelings, emotions, thoughts, and will.

Objectives

1. The endocrine gland system stands high in the hierarchy of the physical systems.

2. These glands also form a link between the body and mind.

3. The function of the glands can be improved by making the mind balanced and calm.

The structure

According to modern science, the pituitary gland is the master gland that controls the functions of all other endocrine glands.

The seven sets of endocrine glands are as follows:

1. Sex glands – testes in the male and ovaries in the female

2. Adrenal glands – support the functions of the kidneys, bones, bone marrow, and spine

3. Pancreas – helps to maintain the entire digestive system, including blood sugar and body temperature; also responsible for hypoglycemia (low blood sugar) or hyperglycemia (diabetes). Deficiency of the pancreas leads to the craving of certain foods, such as sweets.

4. Thymus – governs the heart and circulatory system; it is located between the two nipples in the chest

5. Thyroid – controls growth

6. Pituitary – the master gland (according to modern science), located at base of the skull, controls all other endocrine glands indirectly

7. Pineal – located at the level of the third eye in the center of the head

Endocrine glands have a major impact on our physical, mental, spiritual well being.

Unique concept of Taoism

Stephen T. Chang, MD, in his book *Complete System of Self Healing, Internal Exercises* states that sex glands are sources of energy for all other glands. He also states that the pituitary gland is the seat of memory, wisdom, intelligence, and thought. Modern scientists may not agree with this concept.

Dr. Chang further writes that the pineal gland is the seat of psychic and spiritual powers. One interesting note is that only human beings have this gland. This concept is very much like the concept of *chakras* or *kundalini* of Hindu philosophy.

Summary

The endocrine glands control many delicate functions of the body through hormones. Now we also know that the mind has a profound effect on all endocrine glands. Therefore with the help and power of the mind directly or through the endocrine gland system, we can influence most functions of our body.

CHAPTER SEVENTEEN

Mental Health Defined

Since the subject of mental health is so important, let us review its definition: ***Mental health is the ability to deal calmly with the trying and challenging situations of life. It is directly proportional to mental strength and stability.***

Mental health is a product of the human software or psyche. It has three components: mind, intellect, and ego. The hallmarks of the mental stability and strength are:

Mind
a. Balance of mind
b. Presence of mind
c. Balance of emotion

Ego
The realization of the fact that we are all equal or just numbers

Intellect
a. Sharpness
b. Good analytical ability
c. Good insight and foresight

Examples of mentally healthy people are those who constantly try to advance their search for stability and happiness. They are calm and balanced. These people are just short of spiritual health.

The results of mental strength and stability are:

1. One is calm, collected and balanced.
2. One appreciates and enjoys life.

The opposite of mental strength and stability is:

Mind
a. Restless, impatient
b. Nervous, worried, anxious, fearful
c. Negative thoughts
d. Moody, angry

Ego
Either feeling a hero (on the top of the world) or feeling of being a zero, unworthy and hopeless

Intellect
a. Dull or not sharp
b. Poor analytical ability
c. Poor judgment, poor insight, and foresight

Here is a real life example: Let's say a man loses his job, house, spouse, wealth, or gets insulted, and so on. Now appreciate how the person of mental strength and stability would react differently from the person with mental weakness and instability in this situation:

One with mental strength and stability:

1. Will try to understand what has happened
2. Will plan for tomorrow or and the future
3. Most importantly will not give in or lose himself

In contrast, an individual with mental weakness and instability:

1. May get sad or angry
2. May get depressed or hysterical
3. May blame himself and others
4. May want to kill someone or himself
5. May lose himself

The key message

If you are a mentally strong and healthy person, nothing is a surprise. You understand that life can be like a maze, where everything is possible. In other words, a person of good mental stability/mental health will be less easily moved or affected with any situation or circumstance in life (positive and negative).

After thoroughly understanding the definition of mental health, now let us proceed with the study of the human software/ human psyche.

CHAPTER EIGHTEEN

Human Psyche / Human Software

What lies before us, and what lies
behind us are very tiny matters
compared from what lies within us.

—*Ralph Waldo Emerson*

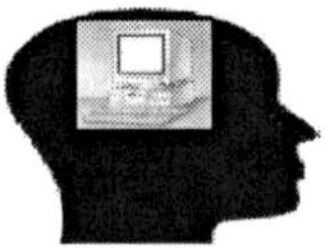

Recently computer technology has taken over everything in life. However in the universe everything is computerized, programmed, and automated from its inception. Our brain is a typical example of that. It is the most sophisticated computer on Earth, and it may never be possible to duplicate it.

You all know that the real value of the computer lies in its software. In this chapter, we will study the software of the human brain, the most sophisticated computer. The software of our brain is also known as our psyche. From now on I shall use the word software of the human brain and human psyche interchangeably.

The role of our psyche (human software) in keeping us not only young but also healthy and happy is more important than any other single element known to us. Everyone is the product of their own psyche (software).

The psyche or software of each person is quite different. The psyche of a sad, poor, and a depressed person can quite different or even the opposite of a happy, prosperous, and blissful person.

There are six billion people in this world. Everybody thinks, acts, and behaves differently. Everybody has a different face, different voice, different fingerprints, and different lines on the palm of their hands, different DNA, and so on. The difference can be so great and profound that they may think, say, and act in a very opposite manner in similar situations. It is all due to a different psyche or software.

You must have observed that some people are happy being wealthy; others are happy as beggars. Some look at a subject or read and can remember it for their lives, while others cannot learn a word. Some strive to reach the top; others are very contented with menial jobs. Some constantly try to improve; others die as they were born. Some love to cheat, steal and rob and yet feel proud of their actions. (It may sound strange but it's true.) Then there are others who enjoy giving, helping, and taking pride in their humane acts.

But the best, most useful, and most practical fact is that it is possible to change your psyche (software) for your benefit.

Objectives

1. We are the product of our psyche (software).

2. We can change our psyche (software) by just changing our thought process.

Introduction

We must understand that the human psyche is responsible for shaping our lives. It is subtler than DNA; hence the psyche is the cause and the body is the effect. This is in keeping up with the cause and effect phenomenon. There's a saying in India: "Jaisa Raja Taisi Praja." It means as is the king, so is the public.

Definition

The psyche can be defined as to outwit, to outguess, to analyze beforehand or to prepare oneself psychologically. It also means to excite. Psyche is not just the mind only, as sometimes misinterpreted.

Understanding the human psyche (software)

In order to simplify this, let us ask ourselves two questions:

1. What are the three elements of the human psyche?
2. How does the psyche affect our lives?

Human psyche (software): Its three elements

According to psychoanalytical theory, the psyche consists of three elements: mind, intellect, and ego. This will be discussed in details in subsequent chapters, but to give you a brief overview, let me mention some salient features:

<u>Mind</u>

The mind is the decision-making element of the human psyche. The mind itself has three components: thoughts (positive or negative), feelings or emotions, and will or determination. Swami Vivekanand states that the mind is such a powerful element that: "Whether one shall live in heaven or hell will also depend upon the decision of the mind."

Intellect

Intellect means knowing. We know what the value of a person would be without intellect, knowledge, and wisdom. Ignorance is one of the most important causes of most suffering and misery. Conversely knowledge and wisdom is the cause of happiness. It is the intellect that can convert a primitive man into an evolved human being, and a human into the divine.

Ego

Ego is self-identification from others. Ego is the essential element for one's creation, development, and sustenance. The balanced ego is the cause of health. On the contrary, ego off-balance can be the cause of pain, misery, suffering, depression, mania, and so on.

How the psyche affects our lives

We know that we are the product of our psyche. The person with a primitive psyche lives the life of a primitive person, and the person with the highest developed psyche lives the life of a highly developed person.

Human psyche differs from person to person: Why?

The human psyche is the result of several variable factors: (a) different level of development of the mind, intellect, and ego; (b) upbringing of childhood and *sanskara*; (c) knowledge and/or education; (d) life experiences; and (e) experiences of past lives (if you believe in reincarnation).

Test: Do I have a good psyche?

Mind

I am fairly balanced in my mood and emotions.	Y/N
My mind is fairly calm and balanced.	Y/N
I usually make good decisions.	Y/N

Intellect

I have good analytic ability.	Y/N
I can think with clarity.	Y/N
Usually I don't have to repent for my decisions.	Y/N

Ego

I understand that we are all created equal.	Y/N
My dealing with others is good.	Y/N

If you have answered most of the questions with yes, then you have a good psyche. Congratulations!

How to improve the psyche (software) for a healthier, happier life

Our psyche or software consists of three elements: mind, intellect, and ego. Now let us discuss how we can change, modify, and/or improve these three elements for a better, healthier, and happier life. Let us continue…

Part I: Ego

Ego is the first element of the human software or psyche. It is an essential ingredient of one's creation and sustenance. However, for mental well being and happiness, the balance of ego (or even abnegation of ego) is essential.

When one's ego is balanced, then one no longer remains a victim of being belittled, disrespected or ignored, and one feels at ease in most situations. All great souls (people) are such examples.

Let us try to understand how the imbalance of the ego can affect one's life. People with high self-esteem or ego are angry, impatient, and bossy. People with low self-esteem or ego are sad and depressed. Worst are those who swing between highs and lows (manic/depressive).

You might have noticed that people with high self-esteem walk as if they are very special, elite, and on the top of the world. They believe that they are the best. How can anybody be better than them? In contrast, people with low self-esteem hide and are afraid to be seen. They believe they do not deserve much in this life. They are suppressed and are even taken advantage of. Both types of people are victims of the imbalance of ego.

Objectives

1. To understand that ego is an important ingredient for one's creation and sustenance

2. To provide a deeper understanding of one's real worth (ego)

3. To understand that balanced or the abnegation (getting rid of) of ego can contribute towards a healthy and blissful living.

4. To learn how to balance one's ego

Definition

Ego is the consciousness of an individual being, in distinction from other self. It is one of the three divisions of the human psyche in psychoanalytic theory. According to *The Oxford Dictionary*, ego is the person's sense of self-esteem or self-importance. It is the part of the mind that meditates between conscious and subconscious and is responsible for reality testing and a sense of personal identity.

Role of ego in the creation of the self

Here I would like to quote from *Bhagavad Gita*: "The eight elemental qualities that enter into all created life from atom to man are: (1) earth (2) water (3) fire (4) air (5) ether (6) sensory mind (*manas*) (7) intelligence (Buddha) and (8) individuality or ego (*ahamkara*).

Imbalanced ego: A cause of suffering

Ego can be measured by self-esteem and self-importance. I have mentioned earlier that although ego is essential for one's creation and existence, ego off-balance, whether high or low, is both equally detrimental and can cause misery and suffering. Let us observe how both types of people suffer:

Behavior of people with low self-esteem/ self-importance/ego

They are nervous, isolated, and behind. They stay behind everywhere at home, in school, at work, and in life. They are neither high achievers nor happy. They lack confidence. They are afraid to take initiative. They fear taking on new projects because of the fear of failure.

Causes of low self-esteem

1. Genetics

2. Degradation by parents, siblings, classmates, spouses on an ongoing basis

3. Multiple and continuous negative outcomes and failures

4. Lack of spiritual growth

People with high self-esteem/self-importance/ego

Vedas says: "Oh, man, you are divine!" This is a beautiful phrase for uplifting mankind. It encourages the person to be divine, so that their actions would be divine. Unfortunately people with inflated egos read this halfway. They read that they alone are divine, and none else.

Many miseries arise due to the ignorance that one is superior and better or more important than all others. This is pure ignorance. It is only in one's head. It is somewhat natural that people think that they are better and their culture is better, but people with inflated egos not only think they are the best, but they also are sure that is the case. This creates a problem.

Behavior of people with inflated egos

1. Self-praise

2. Selfishness

3. Prejudiced way of thinking

4. Insistence on being first everywhere

5. Insistence on winning, irrespective of right and wrong

6. Lack of perception of right and wrong, due to lack of insight.

7. Fault-finding of others

8. Ill treatment of others, due to superiority complex

9. Attention-seeking behavior: I demand, I need, I must

10. Poor listening habits, poor learner, due to the misbelief that they know it all.

11. Attempts to change others to their liking (Remember that no one can change us, thank God. In return I shall happily accept that I will not be able to change others either. Swami Dayanand Ji of Saylorsburg, PA writes in the collection of his speeches, "In early years of my life I used to think I could change people, but that was then.")

Suffering of people with inflated egos

1. They feel insulted. People with high egos expect respect and honor from others and want others to follow them. This is not in vogue in society, so they feel belittled, dishonored, and disrespected. This makes them angry or even depressed.

2. They are more likely to fail. They take projects out of reality and expectation. While taking projects, they do not see the negative aspects of the venture and hence are not prepared well.

3. They are blind to their own weaknesses.

4. They are quick to point out the weaknesses of others.

5. They judge others, and their remarks often result in arguments or fights.

Reasons for inflated ego

1. Genetics

2. Poor and improper upbringing, lack of love, support and suppression

3. The reverse, i.e., fulfillment of every desire, right or wrong

4. Multiple and continuous successes and positive outcomes

5. Lack of mental and spiritual growth

Real examples of ego off-balance

Following are the three examples of ego off-balance. Just observe and analyze. These are real life cases, but the identities are not disclosed.

Example #1

A husband leaves the wife because she is arrogant, pushy, and controlling. Now the wife is suffering. She states, "If my husband will come and ask for forgiveness, I will forgive him." When I interviewed the husband, I asked him about his reaction. He replies, "I'm so glad to be out of that hell. Why would I go back?"

Example #2

A brother and sister had a fight, big-time. They have not spoken to each other in fifteen years. I asked the sister, "Why you don't compromise?" Her reply was, "Why should I? Let him suffer." I asked her brother, and his response was, "I am much better off now than before."

Example #3

A mother and daughter had a fight and have not spoken for years. The mother states "Look at the mistakes of my daughter. She doesn't realize that her grandchildren are not getting my love. How stupid is my daughter?" I asked the daughter for her opinion. She replied, "My mother is so arrogant that she does not understand that she is missing the love of her grandchildren."

You can see how ego blinds individuals of their own weaknesses.

Evaluation of one's ego

A. Sincere evaluation of the self or ego
B. Test

Sincere evaluation: a concept
Evaluation of one's self is also complex. The evaluation of the self can vary from zero to hero, depending upon several factors. Self-evaluation can be performed in one of the following manners:

A. Evaluation by oneself
B. Evaluation by others
C. Zero in on all factors
D. Meta-analysis

Self-evaluation
Self-evaluation could vary greatly from zero to hero based upon:

1. Self-esteem
2. Insight

The higher the self-esteem one has, the higher their self-evaluation will be. On the contrary, the lower the self-esteem one has, the lower their self-evaluation will be. The better the insight one has, the more sincere their self-evaluation will be. Such is the importance of insight.

Do you agree?

Evaluation by others
It may be as complex as self-evaluation, because others can also evaluate you from zero to hero, based upon many factors or situations. Let us explore how that can be.

1. One can be hero in the opinion of their mother, small children, and friends in need.

2. One can be zero according to their adversaries, friends, and spouse, or even their own teenage children after a quarrel or an argument.

Final evaluation: Zero in all of the facts

The best way to evaluate your ego is to do the following:

1. Make a list of all your strengths and weaknesses.

2. Make a list of anything good that you have heard about you from anyone including your friends, parents, and relatives.

3. Make a list of anything bad or negative that you have heard about you from anyone including your friends, relative, and adversities.

4. Zero in on all of the facts together. Probably you will come to a fairly correct analysis.

Meta-analysis: Where would you place yourself?

1. The world population is approximately six billion, and you are one of them.

2. ***Think about how many people sincerely and truly love you***. I have found an easy formula to figure that out. The number of the people who really love you is usually equal to the number of people whom you really care for and love in your heart (minus your children and parents).

3. What would be your status if you lost your job or your license to practice, whatever that field it may be?

4. Did you ever think what would happen to you after retirement?

5. Did you ever think what will happen in your old age or who will take care of you?

6. I was told the world did exist before me (as if I did not know) and that it will continue to exist after I go.

7. Everything is transitory in nature, including you and me.

8. Do you see ego in great people like Jesus Christ, Lord Ram, Lord Krishna, Maharishi Dayanand, Lord Buddha, and Mahatma Gandhi?

Remember Mahatma Gandhi and Lord Buddha used to say we are all zero. What is your opinion? Were they not correct? They were enlightened souls with foresight and insight.

Tests: Is my ego balanced?

Test #1

I think
I am not somebody special. Y/N

I am not at the bottom of the ocean. Y/N

I believe
We are all created equal. Y/N

I am aware
The world existed before me and will continue to exist after me, as usual. Y/N

The world may not change after my death. Y/N

I may be hero today, but someday I may be zero. Y/N

I understand even the ugliest, the homeless, the poorest, and the fool is also being loved by someone and may be the dearest to someone. Y/N

The most brilliant, most handsome, and richest person can be a cause of anger and hate for someone. Y/N

I know that
I may think I am the best, but others may not agree. Y/N

Buddha and Mahatma Gandhi used to say we are all zero. Y/N

If most or all of your answers are yes, then your ego is balanced. Otherwise you may need to read this chapter again. Please do not hesitate to do a second reading. No one is watching you!

Test # 2

If you sincerely understand and believe the following, then you are wise and have a balanced ego: We are equal and just numbers, irrespective of social status, knowledge, education, and power. Nobody is perfect in this universe. Everybody has good and bad qualities. I am no exception to this rule.

An eye-opening true story

The following is a true incident for your insight and consideration. Once I witnessed a poor maid being abused by a rich man. I cannot forget the words of the poor maid, "I understand I am poor. I understand I am uneducated. I understand that you can kick me out of the house. But I am also a human being. I also have a mind. I also have a heart. I also have a husband and two children who love me as much as your children love you. And lastly God is witness to what is happening now. Someday He will listen to me."

After hearing this, the man was taken aback. His face turned pale and he became wonderstruck. He realized what he was doing!

Have you witnessed such incidents in your life? I will bet you have. They may not be exactly of the same nature, but these things do happen in this world. Think about it.

The lesson

It is important to understand the harsh truth that we are just numbers. This we are learning painfully with the advancement of computer technology. We are one of the six billion people on Earth (we are counting only Earth, not the whole universe). Whether we call ourselves hero or zero, it is all in our head. It is just for our own satisfaction.

Mahatma Gandhi and Lord Buddha vocalized, advocated, and practiced the abnegation of ego. They were the spiritual masters. The day we come to the realization or the light dawns upon us that we are all equal and interdependent, not superior or inferior, not better or worse, not less important or more important, life can change. Ignorance and darkness can disappear to a great extent. Happiness will begin to come home.

Practical suggestion for balancing the ego

To people with low self-esteem

We are all created equal. In God's family everybody is loved and cared for. Everybody contributes in its own way. I'm sure you have some quality that others don't possess. Wake up and rise! You may not be the best in one field but you may be better than others in something else! You still have plenty of time to grow and improve. If you have been given this precious life, you must have done something good to get it. Take advantage of it. The time is now.

To people with high self-esteem

You are a poor evaluator of yourself and others. Take the test to see how important you are in the book of others. Don't stay focused only on your positive qualities, but also look at your negative hidden qualities. You don't have to make those public. Everybody has negative and positive qualities, and you are no exception. Don't fly; come down to reality and realization, and the sooner the better.

Think how you have contributed to the well-being of others. Great are those who have done something for others. Everybody can do well for themselves; this is just animal instinct. Look at the life of the great gurus, rishi, prophets, masters, saints, and heroes. My friend, wake up!

To those with balanced egos

You have done a great job of balancing the ego. You could shoot for abnegation of ego which is a higher state. Continue to treat everybody equally with love and respect. A balanced ego means a clear understanding that everybody is equal.

To those who have abnegated or renounced their ego

If you have abnegated ego, you are a hero, not a zero. You have realized the absolute truth; therefore you are entitled to bliss. You are an example of great gurus, rishi, and saints. This was the teaching of our spiritual masters.

The key message

In this complex world, you are just a number, irrespective of how good or important you may feel about yourself.

You can just imagine how much importance we give to others, or even to others' suggestions or ideas, no matter how well thought or organized these may be.

Others also think and feel in a similar manner about us, our suggestions, or ideas. So wake up to this realization: "We are no more important than anyone else."

After this realization we no longer will be the victim of being ignored, disrespected, and dishonored. It is a true fact of life, so acknowledge and accept it today and now from your heart and soul. This will improve your life.

Mantra

Today I realize that we are just numbers. We are all created equal. Probably the best way to become a special person is to treat everybody as a special person. All of the greatest people on Earth are known for treating everybody as s special person.

I am Nobody, No Body
I am a self-contained, immortal being and yet nobody, no body…
I'm a doctor highly trained, but without the patients, nobody, no body…
I'm the storekeeper, but without the customers, nobody, no body
I'm a good speaker, but without an audience, nobody, no body…
I'm a great father/mother, but without a child, nobody, no body…
I am a great spouse, but without the other half, nobody, no body…
I thought I was indispensable, but I was told I am nobody, no body…
I am the object, I am the observer, and I am the observation, yet nobody, no body…
I am all in all, yet nobody, no body…
The game of ego is very unique
People who believe are somebody, are nobody no body
And people who realize that they are nobody
Are special and somebody

Hero and Zero is the Game of Life
Hero and zero is one of the games of life
Imbalance of ego causes miseries of life
Balanced ego is the sign of the wise

In one moment I am a hero and the
next moment I am the same zero
It is flakier than the snow dust
It has no body or the shirt
Just like the cloud or the dust
My little boy calls me dad, hero
My teenage son looks at me as zero
My spouse says go to work my hero
In the evening I am the same zero
My friends tell me otherwise
His wife calls him in the morning zero
In the evening when he comes home with the paycheck,
He is her hero

Hero and zero is one of the games of life
Balanced ego is the sign of the wise

At home every little child is a hero
In school they learn to be zero
During school days I am zero
But on the day of graduation I am the hero
Young are everybody's hero
Old are zero and zero
Hero and zero is one of the games of life
Balanced ego is the sign of the wise
The game of hero and zero keep changing
I often get confused and perplexed
But in reality it is clear and simplex
Nobody is hero or zero in real terms
It is a true fact of life
Hero and zero is one of the games of life
Balanced ego is the sign of the wise

I was listening to a sermon
Everybody chooses to play a role
Who cares if it is of a hero or zero?
Hero and zero is one of the game of life
Balance of ego is the sign of the wise

If you understand the stock market,
The game of hero and zero is not much different
I wish to caution you of the true fact
Hero cannot have any peace or rest
Zero enjoys the peace at heart
Hero struggles all his life
Zero is the winner of life
Hero and zero is one of the games of life
Balanced ego is the sign of the wise

Call me Brother, Dr. Pratap or Singhal
But take my sincere advice,
Do not get entangled in the game of hero or zero
To understand this game in reality and sincerity
One has to become zero and zero
One who thinks oneself as a hero, is in reality zero
And one who considers oneself as zero, is

in reality a hero
Hero and zero is one of the games of life
Balanced ego is the sign of thc wisc

Listen to Lord Buddha, Gandhi and the wise
They had understood the game of life
Hero or zero is one of the games of life
Balanced ego is the sign of the wise.

Part II: Intellect

Intellect is the second element of the human software or psyche. You may wish to know what role intelligence plays in keeping you healthy and happy. Intelligence and happiness are directly and proportionately related. An intelligent person is a happy person, and an ignorant person is an unhappy person. It is as simple as that. Any doubt? In a nutshell, happiness = intelligence = happiness.

I personally believe that the real test of the intelligence of an individual is based on the ability to solve the problems of life, and not of math, science, chemistry, biology, computer science, medicine, law or anything else. These later problems only help to pay the bills, but it is the ability to solve the problems of life that can provide ease, comfort, and happiness.

The importance of the intellect and intelligence and their contribution towards health, happiness and/or for a better life is probably too underestimated. It is important to understand that intelligence is the very basis of functioning. It is the intelligent beings who enjoy the life of joy and freedom. They also stay out of trouble or, if they do get into trouble, they know how to get out. Whereas ignorant people suffer not only because they get into trouble easily, but also, once in, they do not know how to get out. In this reference you may also like to know that:

Whereas the ignorant person makes simple things complex,
The intelligent one makes complex things simple.

Whereas the ignorant person gets into trouble,
The intelligent one stays out of trouble.
If ignorance is darkness, then knowledge is light.
If ignorance is confusion, then knowledge is clarity.

If ignorance is groping, then knowledge is the clear path.
If ignorance is dependency, then knowledge is independence and freedom.

If ignorance is suffering, then knowledge is happiness.

We are all gifted with intellect, but it is only the intelligent being that uses it. Going to school and college only educates people enough so that they can pay the bills, however it may or may not make them intelligent. Intelligence does not come from learning. Intelligence comes from the application of the knowledge, especially in reference to life's complexities.

Objective

The purpose of intelligence and learning is not just to make a living; of course that is the natural outcome. But the real purpose of intelligence and true learning is to provide us with a way to enjoy the life of ease, freedom, and happiness.

The importance of intellect

Intellect means to know. Can you imagine the value of a human being without knowledge, without intellect? How would they be different from a primitive being or even an animal?

Is it not true that ignorance is the cause of most miseries and sufferings, whereas wisdom is the cause of happiness and bliss? (Someone once said that education is becoming very expensive, and the other replied jokingly, try living without it!)

Definition

Intellect is the faculty of reasoning and understanding objectively, or one's mental power. Intelligence is the ability to acquire, apply knowledge, and skill, such as analytic ability. Intellect is one of the three elements of the human psyche. Mind and ego are the other two.

Differentiating intellect from related terms

1. Innocence means simplicity and blamelessness of children, or not guilty of crime.

2. Ignorance means lacking knowledge and awareness.

3. Illiteracy means little or no education, or the inability to read or write.

4. Intellect means the power of knowing or capacity for knowing which leads to knowledge.

5. Intelligence means proper application of knowledge and skill, while keeping other factors in balance (emotions, senses, etc.). It is the ability to learn and understand or deal with new trying situations. It is also known as mental acuteness or one's ability to lead a life of freedom and happiness.

6. Knowledge is the information acquired through experience and education.

7. Education is the process of educating or being educated, the theory and practice of teaching.

8. Wisdom is accumulative philosophical and scientific learning, known as insight, good judgment, and wise attitude. Wisdom is also equal to intelligence minus ego.

Dr. Krishnamurti in his book, *Education and Significance of Life*, has given beautiful descriptions of knowledge, intellect, intelligence, and wisdom.

> "It is clear then that merely to cultivate the intellect, which is to develop capacity or knowledge, does not result in intelligence. There is a distinction between intellect and intelligence. Intellect is thought functioning independently of emotions, whereas intelligence is the capacity to feel as well as to reason,

and until we approach life with intelligence, instead of intellect alone, or with emotions alone, no political or educational system in the world can save us from the toils of chaos and destruction. Knowledge is not comparable with intelligence, knowledge is not wisdom. Wisdom cannot be found in books; it cannot be accumulated, memorized, or stored up. Wisdom comes with abnegation of ego (renunciation of the self)."

Intelligence: An essential ingredient

Intelligence is an essential ingredient of each and every thing in this universe from the tiniest, such as an atom, to the largest, such as the universe, and anything in between. As a matter of fact, nothing exists without intelligence, including minerals, plants, animals, and man.

Everything that comes to exist, sustain, and then die is due to its built-in intelligence. Intelligence is responsible for shaping our life, and if used correctly it can be a cause of healthy, happy, and blissful living. For clarification sake, let us appreciate the intelligence of some very basic elements, e.g., the electron, the tiniest component of an atom and the seed in general.

The intelligence of the tiniest electron (part of the tiny atom) knows how to be a part of the atom. It keeps on circling around the nucleus (which consists of protons and neutrons) just to shape the atom and for its own survival, as our Earth revolves around the sun and on its own axis for its own survival and to keep the solar system as one unit.

Behold the intelligence of the seed. If you plant the seed in the ground and water it, it grows. It knows what to imbibe from the ground and how to grow into a plant and then into a tree. It attracts from the earth only those elements that are essential for its growth because of its built-in intelligence. The earth has everything in it, whether it is needed for the growth of that seed or not, but it is up to the seed to decide, what and what not to imbibe from the earth.

Now if we put the same seed into our mouth as food, that seed breaks down into five basic ingredients (five *maha Bhuta*): the ether (heavenly space), air, fire, water and earth; and now those five elements become part of same five elements of our body. Although our body's intelligence plays an important and active role in accepting that seed as food, it is also the intelligence of the seed that helps to facilitate the process.

The same is true when we take medicine, whether it is aspirin, painkillers, penicillin and any other antibiotics, an Ayurvedic preparation, herbal medicines, homeopathic remedies, or any other medicine. The intelligence of that medicine helps us to get better. So the intelligence of everything makes things exist as they are. The same principle applies to all animals, bacteria, insects, and so on.

Emotional intelligence

This is a growing field. It is being recognized more and more that emotions play an extremely important role in our day-to-day life. Religion, sentiments, family bonds, and country bonds have a stronger basis on emotion than intelligence. We often buy things based upon emotion. We buy things because they look or feel good. We do a lot of other things in life, based on emotions.

Emotions may have no logic or rationale, whereas intelligence is based upon logic. You can define emotional intelligence as one's ability to perceive, understand, and manage one's own emotions. People with high emotional intelligence are more aware of their own emotions and also of others. They act in a mature manner and are more balanced and happier in their personal and social life.

People with low emotional intelligence have less control over their emotions. They are less aware of their emotions, as well as of others.

Relatively speaking, these people are unhappier in their personal and social life, compared to people with high emotional intelligence.

For in-depth study on the subject, I refer you to the book titled *Emotional Intelligence* by Daniel Goleman.

Knowledge

Knowledge is vast; it is as vast as the universe. In this reference, let us study the types of knowledge, the source of knowledge, the method of learning, and also why people don't learn.

Types of knowledge

<u>Study of nature</u>

This includes all materialistic sciences, e.g., medicine, law, engineering, math, physics, chemistry, astrology, biology, astronomy, accounting, and so on. Swami Vivekanand states that scientific knowledge does not contribute to mental health.

<u>Metaphysical and spiritual knowledge</u>

This knowledge is essential for mental health and stability. It includes knowledge about self (soul) and/or God. This involves study of the *Bible*, the Vedas, the Upanishad, the Gita, the Koran, and other religious scriptures, or a deep thorough inquiry into one's life. Such knowledge, if read and understood from the heart and soul, sheds light on the truth or the path of happiness, path of higher evolution, path of freedom, and happiness.

<u>Knowing self or knowledge of self</u>

The importance of this knowledge supersedes all other knowledge. Without knowledge of self, you are incomplete and dependent; hence you may be vulnerable to most suffering and miseries of life. This knowledge may be hard to learn by alone and may require the help of a guru, teacher, or spiritual master.

In order to understand yourself, you must understand the following:

A. How to live the life of a child

B. How to live the life of a student

C. How to live the life of a married person, if you decide to get married. This is the toughest part of life where one has to play multiple roles of a parent, spouse, and son/daughter and also as a part of the community.

D. How to live happily when children leave home for their independent life

E. How to live with or without a spouse in later years of life. This could be tough and challenging at times. Not only this, it is the age when one may need his or her spouse more than ever before.

F. How to understand life and the purpose of life. Probably this is a single most important secret in understanding the self.

G. What you need to accomplish in your life intellectually, spiritually, emotionally, and so on.

H. You can also gain better understanding of self and life by (1) writing your autobiography and/or obituary, or (2) by studying the stories of great people.

Personal observation/experience

At times I meet people who impress me with their statements. They are calm, patient, and clear in their thought process. They are content and at peace. These people understand life and the meaning of life and hence they are happy. How they got to that stage is a different issue. It could have been their upbringing, their environment, or the cumulative effects of good karma of past lives or spiritual wisdom.

These people may not have seen a school in their lives. They may not be able to add numbers or write a sentence. An average person would call them uneducated. I label them as doctors of life, because they understand life better than many of us. They live more happily than people with many degrees and diplomas.

What is the source of knowledge?

There are different opinions as to what is the real source of all knowledge. According to many religions and beliefs, all knowledge comes through the prophets, the Avatars, the messengers of God.

But according to Vedic philosophy, Buddhist and others beliefs, all knowledge is within us. The religious scriptures—Vedas, Bible, Koran—and the spiritual teachers or gurus just make us aware of knowledge. All great prophets have stressed the fact that anyone can become like them.

The real methods of learning

We can learn in many ways: reading, listening, and discussing, but the best method of learning is inquiry or self-inquiry. No other method matches this one.

The role of intellect and emotions in the learning process

Learning should be from the heart and soul. Just learning from the brain is not very different from programming a computer. All knowledge must integrate emotions and feeling.

Why people don't learn

Many people do not learn because learning requires patience, effort, and hard work. An average person either does not have patience or avoids hard work. They are satisfied with the way they are. Other people don't know that learning is fun, natural, and rewarding.

Intelligence: a cause of happiness

At a basic level

- To make a living
- To learn how to learn
- To have fun
- To develop analytic ability

At a higher level

- To increase mental power and acuity
- To understand the truth
- To prepare for difficult challenges and situations of life
- To understand self and others

At the highest level

- To expand consciousness
- To provide mental and spiritual strength>independence> freedom>happiness
- To make you humble

Sequence summary

1. Intellect leads to knowledge.
2. Knowledge leads to learning.
3. Learning in balance with emotions and feeling leads to intelligence.
4. Intelligence minus ego means wisdom.
5. Wisdom makes one>free>happy blissful.

Quotations/sayings about knowledge and intelligence

Swami Yogananda Parmahansa

The best purpose of education is to develop personality.

Swami Vivekanand

- The personality of the teacher is based on experience and not just pure knowledge.

- Philosophers and prophets are quite different. Both have extensive knowledge. Philosophers cannot influence people because their knowledge lacks experience. But prophets have the ability to influence the public because of the experience they have.

- Small things don't affect a wise person. The greater and wiser a person is, the less likely they will be affected by things or situations (good and bad, positive and negative) and by other people.

- Never say that our forefathers knew so much. What is stopping you from learning? Are you giving up?

- Intellect and analysis are very powerful. After a deep analysis, infinite becomes finite, and finite becomes infinite.

- He also writes that:

  We want that education by which
  Character is formed,
  Strength of mind is increased.
  The intellect is expanded,
  And by which one can stand on one's own feet.

<u>Vedas</u>

1. Oh God, guide our intelligence and bestow sweetness in our speech.

2. Grant us knowledge not to insult anyone.

3. Grant us intelligence so that we can keep the company of the learned people.

4. Scientific knowledge does not contribute to mental health. To study knowledge, for the sake of knowledge, in the search of truth is known as Janan Yoga. This knowledge leads to freedom of the soul.

5. Vedas states that "all the knowledge is within us."

<u>Swami Dayanand of Saylorsburg, PA</u>

The purpose of learning is to create awareness. Everything is here in this universe. A good teacher makes us see what is here.

<u>Lord Krishna</u>

Knowledge is superior to action.

Test

Am I an intelligent being?

Study the questions and try to answer them. The answers may be kept confidential: The test is only for insight, not to judge you.

<u>Personal</u>

I usually think before I speak.	Y/N
I am calm while making decisions.	Y/N
I try to make complex things simple.	Y/N
I usually make decisions for which I don't have to repent.	Y/N
I do not get into the problem easy, but if I do, I don't get sad or despair, and solve the problem calmly.	Y/N
I strive for constant improvement on daily basis.	Y/N
Now I have come to the realization that I am not more important than anyone else.	Y/N
I am a happy person.	Y/N

<u>Interpersonal</u>

I avoid arguments.	Y/N
I don't criticize others.	Y/N
I do not try to change others. I understand that if no one could change me, then how could I change anyone else? Even the greatest people on Earth could not change anyone.	Y/N

If you have answered most or all questions with yes, then you are an intelligent being. Congratulations! If you did not, do not be discouraged. Please re-read the chapter.

The final clue of intelligence

If you are happy or at least stay calm in difficult situations of life, then you are entitled to be labeled an intelligent being. However if you get sad, angry, miserable, and become unhappy for long periods of time, then you should not call yourself an intelligent being.

Test of wisdom (steady wisdom)

Wisdom is a higher state than intelligence. A wise person is calmer, more stable, balanced, and happier, because he has given up his ego. Best of all, wisdom makes one humble. Lord Krishna makes a statement in reference to wisdom in the book titled *Bhagavad Gita.* Following is a part of a dialogue between Arjuna (the pupil) and the Lord Krishna (the guru, the lord):

ARJUNA ASKED:

What is the description of the man of steady wisdom who is merged in the super-conscious state, O Kesava? How does one of steady wisdom speak? How does he sit? How does he walk?

THE BLESSED LORD SAID:

"When a man casts away, O Partha, all desires of the mind and is satisfied in the self alone by the self, then he is said to be one of steady wisdom. He whose mind is not agitated by sorrow, nor excited by joy, which is free from passion, fear and anger, he is called a sage of steady wisdom. He who is everywhere without attachment, whatever happens, fair or foul, who neither rejoices nor hates, his wisdom is well established. When, again, as a tortoise draws in on all sides its limbs, he withdraws his senses from objects, then his wisdom is well established."

Benefits

Helps you understand:

1. Yourself in wholeness and thoroughness (See Chapter 4)

2. Your life as a whole, not in parts

3. All issues as a whole, not in parts

4. Yourself as a happier person in face of thousands of trivial issues of life

5. How to realize and meditate on the ultimate goal of life

6. How to stay focused on goals in life

7. That everybody is okay. People are because that's how they are. No one can change you, nor can you change anyone else. Don't waste your time and energy.

8. How to take pride in simplifying issues and life. Ignore and filter small issues for the sake of comfort and joy of life.

The key message

If you are not enjoying a life of ease, freedom and happiness, then you should not call yourself an intelligent person, irrespective of what else you may have achieved in the form of education, diplomas, degrees, wealth, social status, and so on. You need to think and rethink how to make it happen.

Mantra **(Recite it on a daily basis for thirty days.)**

Now I understand that happiness is a product of intelligence. Now I can appreciate that happy people are intelligent, and intelligent people are happy. I shall also stay calm, relaxed, and deal with all difficult situations and circumstances intelligently, whether this is the result of my own fault or even of others.

Freedom and Happiness are the Symbols of the Wise

Intelligence is the basis of life
Ignorant is lost in life
Misery and pain belongs to the unwise
Freedom and happiness is symbol of the wise…

Art, math, chemistry, and physics or any other skill
It only helps to pay the bills
Understanding the self is the secret of life
Misery and pain belongs to unwise
Freedom and happiness is symbol of the wise…

Pain and suffering are part of everybody's life
Intelligent one understands this fact
Ignorant could not have this depth
Intelligent is calm in most situations and act
Ignorance is often confused and perplexed
Misery and pain belongs to unwise
Freedom and happiness is symbol of the wise…

Ignorant one gives up after the first attempt
Intelligent does not mind extra attempts
The results are counted only of the final attempt
Edison took the advantage of this fact
He continued to make attempts after attempts
Till he completed his final project
Misery and pain belongs to unwise
Freedom and happiness is symbol of the wise…

Ignorant often makes wrong decision
Intelligence comes to right conclusion
Ignorant gropes in the dark
Intelligence knows his path
Misery and pain belongs to unwise
Freedom and happiness is symbol of the wise…

Call me Doctor, Brother, Pratap or Singhal
Take it as a warning or advice
If you are unhappy, you should not claim
yourself intelligent or wise

If you are wise, then nothing should be a surprise
You should know that happiness is the mission of life,
Misery and pain belongs to unwise
Freedom and happiness is symbol of the wise…

So far I have discussed two important elements of human psyche (software): ego and intellect. Now I shall discuss the third element of the human psyche: the mind.

Part III: The Mind

The mind is the third and probably the most powerful element of the human software or human psyche. Remember your mind is magical, and it can do wonders. Its role is like that of a governor, manager, or CEO. You also know that your life is the product of the decisions and choices that we make. So why not make up your mind right now, right this minute, what type of life would you wish to lead?

Now read the following mantra **three times** from your heart and soul before going any further into the study of the mind:

> *From this very moment I shall live the life of health and happiness. This is my decision. This is my commitment to myself. I shall work on it throughout my life with my heart and soul. No if, ands or buts.*

This mantra looks very simple, yet it is very powerful. It can change your life. It is all within the power of your mind. You are today what you wanted to be yesterday. Whether you are a clerk, businessman, accountant, attorney, doctor, nurse or anything else, it is because you made that decision some time ago. Going one step further, tomorrow or in the near future you will be what you decide today. If you make this decision that you will live the life of a healthy and happy person from today on, you will do everything possible to achieve that goal. Nothing can or will prevent you from achieving that goal. Think it over. Take a pause. It is your call!

The next time you meet a happy person ask what makes them happy, most likely you will hear only one answer at least most of the time: "It is my decision. I have problems like everyone else, but I do not let them bother me."

To understand the power of the mind, read, think, and analyze the following two quotations:

"If you think you will live in heaven for the rest of your life, you will. But if you think you will live in hell for the rest of your life, you will." —*Swami Vivekanand.*

"If you think you can do it, you are right. However, if you think you cannot do it, you are also right." —*Henry Ford*

Whatever role our mind plays in keeping us healthy and or happy can also be understood by a simple day-to-day experience. Two people with similar education, background, living under the same roof, in similar situations, and at the same time can have a very different life based upon the perception of their mind.

In a difficult situation, the people with a well balanced and focused mind will analyze the situations and facts, and then do their best to change whatever can be changed, but will also accept whatever is not within their control and will then put themselves at ease; whereas the people with an unbalanced mind may have a problem in analyzing or dealing with the same problem or situation. They may become the victim of the situation and/or may become sad, miserable, and depressed. Such is the power of the mind. Okay so far?

Objectives

1. The mind is an extremely powerful element. Its role is that of manager or CEO. It runs our life.

2. If you wish to lead the life of health and happiness, you have to make such a decision and a commitment; then the rest of the things shall fall into place by itself.

3. A healthy, calm, balanced mind is the key to a healthy and happy life.

Introduction

"We are what we think we are." All of our thinking or thoughts have their origin in the mind. In other words directly or indirectly we are the product of the mind. In this reference, Swami Vivekanand used to say: "Mind can move the mountains and dry the oceans."

Furthermore we must be very clear that we are the product of our thoughts, and thoughts are the products of our mind. Think and meditate on this aphorism. Breathe deeply! Take a pause! Please do not rush. This information is too important.

In the Sanskrit language, the mind is called *mana* where the "a" is silent. I wonder if the word "man" comes from the Sanskrit word *mana*.

Thoughts: Products of the mind

Analyze and understand the following to appreciate how thoughts are the forerunners of life:

If you believe that life is nothing but pain and misery, then you are correct. But conversely if you believe life is joy and happiness, then you are also correct.

If you believe that you are a victim and helpless, then you are correct. Conversely if you believe that you are in charge and the master of your life, then you are also correct.

If you believe that you are surrounded by enemies everywhere and have to be careful at every step, then you are correct. But conversely if you believe that you are surrounded by friends and dear ones, then you are also correct.

If you believe that you are the victim of life and are unfortunate, then you are correct. But conversely if you believe that life is an opportunity which you received after millions of lives, then you are also correct.

An interesting true story

This story is about some naughty students who wanted an evening off from class. They made a plan. Each of them decided that they would tell their teacher independently that he was looking sick. The story goes like this:

This teacher used to have an evening class for students who needed extra help. One day as the teacher arrived in class, the students launched their plan. It worked in the favor of the students because the teacher was looking a little tired that day. He must have had rough day at work and/or school. Now the first student asked the teacher, "Sir, are you okay? You do not look normal."

The second student said, "Sir, you look a little ill." Then the third classmate said, "Sir, would you like me to bring you some fever medicine or tea before you start the class?"

Before fourth student opened his mouth, the teacher said, "Stop it! I know what you are going to say. I agree with all of you that today I am not well. I think you should take the evening off. I need some rest."

Mission accomplished. Do you appreciate how the mind can affect your life and/or the lives of others?

Definition

As defined by the dictionary, the mind is part of the individual that feels, perceives, thinks, wills, and especially reasons. Of the human psyche, the mind is one of three components; the other two are the intellect (to know) and ego (self-identification).

Please also understand what the mind is not. It is not the soul or senses or the spirit as misinterpreted at times. The mind should never be confused with the brain. The brain is a physical organ; one can touch, feel, and see it, whereas the mind is a metaphysical element or part of the human software; at best one can perceive it.

Attributes of the mind

Imagination

You know imagination is a function of the mind. Albert Einstein used to say "imagination is more important than intelligence."

The mind can imagine anything and everything. By imagination, in one moment one can become a king and the next moment a beggar. In one minute one can be on the top of the mountain, second moment at the bottom of the ocean.

The imagination of the mind is such that man has created even God in his own image, which is why all of the idols of God look like either man or woman. Swami Vivekanand states that if you ask the dog to portray God, the dog will portray God as a bigger dog, and not a human being. And if you ask a rat to portray a God, the rat will portray God as a bigger rat, and not a human being.

Speed of the mind

The mind travels faster than anything known to mankind. Light travels at the rate of 186,000 miles per second, but the mind is millions and billions times faster than that. In one second, the mind can take one to the moon and the next second to Mars.

Power

Remember the common proverb "The mind can move mountains and dry the ocean," speaking metaphorically. Once again I would remind you of the quotation from Swami Vivekanand, "If you think you will live in heaven, you will."

Lord Krishna states in *Bhagavad Gita* (the song divine) that the mind is as powerful as the wind. He also used to state: "Anybody who can conquer their mind, can conquer the world."

The great people of the world have used the power of the mind to succeed in their lives; so can we. Agree?

The mind: its three components

Thoughts

We know that the mind is busy, imaginative, fast, and creative. The mind is the mother of all thoughts. The human mind creates a thought every one to one-and-a-half seconds. That is equal to approximately 60,000 to 80,000 thoughts per day. Probably that is the reason why the mind is so busy, traveling, fleeting, and restless. Of course 90 to 95 percent of thoughts are just repetitive and probably not of much value.

Feeling, sensitivity, and emotions

Emotions and feelings are some of the most important components of life. Lack of emotions and feelings can make one inhuman and cruel, and bring one to the lowest level. It is important to understand that emotions may have no logic or rationale in the real scientific terms; therefore one must keep a check on their emotions with intelligence or suffer immensely.

Will

The will is the faculty that makes a person decide or initiate action. The stronger the will and determination, the better one's ability will be to initiate action and carry it to its full execution and success. One of the important reasons why people with a weak will do not succeed is that either they do not initiate any new project or if they do, they leave it without completion.

How the mind functions

Functioning of the mind can be understood in two ways: at a global level and at the cellular level. At the global level, the mind gathers all of the information from every possible source, analyzes it, comes to a decision, and then carries it to execution.

At the cellular level, Swami Vivekanand writes:

> "[The] mind operates by perception and impulsion. For instance the rays of light enter into the eyes, or [are] carried by the nerves to the brain, and still I do not see the light. The brain then conveys the impulse to the mind but yet I do not see the light. [The] mind then reacts and the light flashes across the mind. The mind reaction is impulsion, and as a result the eye perceives the object. This is at the cellular level."

I'm sure if Swami Ji had spoken further, he would have said that even the mind cannot see without the soul. The mind is useless without soul. Therefore to see an object, one needs to have an object, light, eyes, brain, mind, and finally soul.

The functions of the mind

The mind has multiple and varied functions, the most important being:

1. The mother of all thoughts; we are the product of our thoughts.

2. Memory: the first step of memory is the learning process. Learning depends on the focus, concentration, and the interest of the mind. (Our subconscious mind is the mother seat of all memories.)

3. Concentration, a function of a good and healthy mind.

4. Decision-making, the most important function of the human mind, because our life is a product of the decisions and choices that we make.

5. Healing. Our body is the reflection of our mind and subconscious mind. Our mind and subconscious mind are the reflections of our thoughts and belief system. So by changing our thoughts and belief system, we could change our mind and subconscious mind, thereby

our body. This is the principle of healing with hypnosis and/or meditation.

How decisions affect our life

Our life is based on the decisions we make. An important decision can put us in the driver's seat, and conversely one bad decision can put us out of the loop. Such is the value of a decision. Any important decision, right or wrong, can have a positive or negative effect on our personal life, family life, community life, or even for generations to come.

Decision-making: a process

We have discussed before that the mind is the decision-making faculty of the human psyche. Decisions are made after the following considerations:

- Information available or presented
- Desires of the senses: eye (vision), ear (hearing), nose (smell), tongue (taste), and skin (touch)
- Emotions and feelings
- Intellectual analysis
- Template created by the subconscious mind (the reservoir of information of all the experiences of this life and the experiences of past lives, if you believe in reincarnation)
- Inner voice of the soul/spirit, a very important component

How to improve the decision-making ability:

Keep the mind calm and even (it increases awareness).

1. Keep the mind focused. (See Chapter 46)
2. Make a list of all of the facts, positive and negative, and weigh them against each other.

3. Be more objective (intellectual) than emotional or subjective.

4. Try to appreciate and/or analyze others' points of view. (This factor alone can significantly boost one's decision-making ability.)

5. A global understanding of the issue as a whole, ignoring the trivial elements. This is also one of the important guiding elements.

6. Lastly but probably the best point to consider is what is beneficial for all.

The balanced and/or healthy mind vs. unbalanced and/or unhealthy mind: A study

In order to appreciate the effect of balanced and unbalanced mind on life, it is best to study the people with corresponding attributes that follow:

People with a balanced and healthy mind have the following qualities:

Balanced nature

Probably this is the single most important secret of a person with a healthy mind. A person with a balanced mind is not affected easily or at least not for long by positive or negative situations and outcomes of life.

The path/duties/Dharma

The person with a healthy mind focuses more on the right path, rather than on the results.

Good concentration

These people have good memory, good focus, and clarity of the thought process.

Emotions

People with a healthy mind are quite stable in their emotions and feelings. They do not let their emotions get in the way of decision-making.

Thoughts

Now appreciate the thought process of these people. People with a healthy mind have good and positive thoughts.

- Negative thoughts do not cross their mind, or if they do, they do not last for long.

- Beneficial thoughts: a healthy mind thinks what is good for him or her and for all others.

- Purity of thought: the thoughts are based on facts and truth, not on whims, notions, or beliefs.

Strong will

People with a healthy mind have strong will and determination. Once they make a decision, they carry it to execution.

Avoidance of negativity

People with a healthy mind do not breed the following:

- Fear
- Anxiety and worries
- Anger and hate
- Jealousy
- Bitterness

People with an unbalanced and/or unhealthy mind may have the following negative features:

Mood and emotions

These people are moody by nature. Their behavior is unpredictable. This is the first sure sign of imbalance. They are controlled by feelings and emotions, rather than by objectivity and facts. They can fly off the handle at any time.

Focus

They have no control over their thoughts; rather, their thoughts control them. They lack focus.

Negative and harmful thoughts

They breed negative and harmful thoughts or even miserable thoughts. They get sad, depressed, and find things difficult. They may have delusions and/or paranoia. They might even harm or injure others or even themselves.

Decisions

They may have one or more of the following features:

- They are indecisive: they have difficulty making decisions, because of the lack of clarity, focus, and uncertainty, and hence they procrastinate.

  OR

- They make decisions in a hurry, based on their emotions rather than facts and objectivity. So often they repent or suffer for the decisions and choices that they make.

Will and determination

Their will is weak and determination, poor. They are not sure what they want, so they hesitate to take any initiative or project. If they take on a project, they may leave it in the middle unfinished. This causes failure and frustration.

Other negativity:

- Fear
- Anxieties and worries
- Anger and hate
- Jealousy and greed
- Bitterness
- Getting stuck on little issues

Test

This test is only for better insight and understanding. It provides an opportunity to test the three elements of mind: thoughts, feeling, and will.

Thoughts	
I usually have good, positive, and beneficial thoughts.	Y/N
I do not degrade myself or others.	Y/N
Negative thoughts do not cross my mind, and if they do, I can easily get rid of them.	Y/N
Emotion	
My moods are balanced. (I am not moody.)	Y/N
I have good relationships with most people.	Y/N
I am sincere with people. (Look deep into your heart.)	Y/N
Will and determination	
I have confidence in myself.	Y/N
I have strong will. When I initiate any project, I carry to its execution.	Y/N
General: I am fairly balanced and calm in:	
Ups and downs of life	Y/N
Positive and negative outcomes in life	Y/N
Health and disease	Y/N
Success and failure	Y/N
If I fail or get insulted, I don't grieve for long and bounce right back.	Y/N

If you have answered most or all of the questions with yes, then you are the owner of a healthy and balanced mind. Congratulations! If not, please read this chapter again.

Balance and peace of mind

One must not confuse the two: balance and peace of mind. They are very different entities. Balance of mind is a powerful entity of which you can be proud. Balance of mind is based on inner mental and spiritual strength and good attributes and qualities of the mind, whereas peace of mind is very fleeting and short-lived. Peace of mind is based on temporary external factors and situations, for example buying car insurance, health insurance, house insurance, locking the car, locking the house at night, shutting off the oven, and so on. Going to temple or church and doing prayers can provide only temporary, fleeting peace of mind and not balance of mind.

One must understand that balance of mind is several times more potent and powerful in providing mental and spiritual strength and happiness, than temporary peace of mind.

Practical application

Programming and training the mind for a better life

Now you know the importance of the mind; it basically runs our life. Yet most important is the fact that you can train your mind in the way you like it. Training the mind is your responsibility. You need to train the mind for the following:

- To stay calm and focused. Probably this is one of the top secrets for building a healthy mind. It provides clarity of the thought process. When you get nervous, frightened or angry, you lose focus and clarity and can end up making wrong decisions for which you may have to suffer. You also need to understand that all of these positive and negative situations are temporary in nature, like day and night, summer and winter.

- To stay on the right path. This is more beneficial than focusing on the results. In the long run, you can feel proud and good about it. In order to stress the importance of the right path or duty, Lord Krishna in *Bhagavad Gita* states, "Do your duty and do not think of the result."

- Beneficial and positive thoughts

Our mind is strongly affected by thoughts, positive and negative. We all know that the person who breeds negative thoughts day in and day out also becomes negative. Conversely the person who breeds positive thoughts day in and day out also becomes positive. If you live with a fearful person, you will become fearful, but if you live with a brave person, you also become brave.

I can give you a real life example. One day I was sad and frustrated because of some incident (although this is not my nature). I was listening to the radio and a great master came on, reading from *Bhagavad Gita* something positive, something encouraging. I felt like he was talking to me. My sadness disappeared in no time, and I bounced back.

Just imagine if you could read some positive affirmations on a regular basis for as little as five minutes per day, how much positive impact it could have on your life. Think about it.

Emotions

Emotions can throw you off in the wrong direction; therefore you need to keep them in check. The role of intelligence is extremely important in controlling your emotions.

Healing of the power of the mind

We can use our mind and subconscious mind for healing purposes.

Meditation

The role of meditation in making the mind calm and balanced is more important than any other technique or method. Therefore you must include the practice of meditation on a daily basis. The benefits that you attain from the practice of meditation far outweighs the time spent in meditation. There should not be any question about it.

Reality vs. perception

Generally speaking, you are not so much affected by reality itself but how you perceive or interpret reality. Let us look at some real life examples, and then you will appreciate how the same situation or circumstance can have different, or even opposite effect on an individual.

- All goodness is gone from this world; we are going to ruins
  vs. There are plenty of good things and good people in this world, besides all that is happening.

- I have to work hard or else I will starve and my family will starve; I have no choice. ***vs.***
  The work is life; work is good for the mind and soul. Work is rewarding. Without work we would go crazy.

- I have to work so hard that it is killing me. ***vs***.
  My work is very challenging now I have learned to work more efficiently.

- I am preparing for an exam for a promotion; I hope I don't fail or else I will be kicked out of my job. ***vs***.
  I am preparing for an exam and I hope to do very well. It would be good for me and for the company.

- Mother and son: Dear son, drive carefully so that you don't have another accident. You know that you are accident prone. ***vs***.
  My dear son, drive safely. I know you are a good driver. But there are a lot of careless people on the road. Call me when you get home. I will be thinking about you.

- Why did God give me so much pain, misery, and suffering; there is no let up. ***vs***.
  The pain, misery, and suffering are part and parcel of everybody's life, like joy, health, and happiness or like day and night, and nobody can be exempt from this. This is real life.

- The world is full of thieves and robbers; you have to be careful every step of the way or they will eat you up. ***vs.***
  There are good and bad people everywhere, every community, every ethnic group, at any time in history. Even at times I get bad thoughts.

- I am a victim of life and circumstances. ***vs.***
  My life is full of challenges but I am doing fairly well. Every challenge makes me smarter and better.

- There is so much pain and misery in this world, I wonder if there is anything like God. ***vs.***
  God has given human beings the freedom to act. Everyone is responsible for their own deeds, good and bad. Pleasure and pain are the products of the deeds.

- My friend has been abusing me recently and has been rude to me. I must let off steam at him. ***vs.***
  I need to have a talk with my friend. Why he is acting in this manner? After all, he is my best friend.

- My boss is giving me so much work that is killing me. ***vs.***
  Times are tough and my work load is excessive, but I am lucky I have a job. I can understand the feelings of my boss; he is also being pressured from higher authorities.

These are real examples for your consideration and thoughts.

The key message

A good life is the product of good actions, and good actions are the products of good decisions; and good decisions are the products of positive thoughts and positive feelings; and positive thoughts and positive feelings are the products of a balanced, healthy, and calm mind. We are today what our mind decided to be yesterday. We will be tomorrow what our mind decides today.

Mantra #1 (Recite it on a daily basis for thirty days.)
From this very moment I will live the life of health and happiness. This is my decision. This is my commitment to myself. I will work on it throughout my life from my heart and soul. No if, ands or buts.

Mantra #2 (Recite it on a daily basis for thirty days.)
My mind is strong and pure. It breeds only good, positive, and beneficial thoughts. These thoughts make me stay calm, relaxed, and balanced in all situations and circumstances. Today I am making a decision and a commitment that I shall live the life of health and happiness. No excuses.

Life is a Game; It is a Game of the Mind

Life is a game; it is a game of the mind
If one plays it right, one can win the game of life
If one wins the game
It will be all happy and gain
Or else it will be misery and pain
Life is a game; it is a game of the mind
If one plays it right, one can win the game of life…

Mind is the mighty one
In one moment it can make one king or little beggar
It can dry the pond or wet the land
It can make do anything, which one can imagine
Whether one shall live in hell or heaven
Whether one is getting better or worse
Whether one is surrounded by foe or friends
It is all in the mind and the imagination
Life is a game and is a game of the mind
If one plays it right, one can win the game of life…

The rain could be all joy and pleasure
For the dry land, farmer or the lover
Or it could be all wet and messy for the outer
Is the wind pleasing, refreshing, and cleansing?
Or is it bad for the new seed, or makes one sneeze

It is all in the mind and imagination
Life is a game and is a game of the mind
If one plays it right, one can win the game of life…

Mind is always on the flee/fleet
It can keep one on his/her feet
The wise knew this very fact
They gave little tact,
One must control his/her mind
Or else one can lose one's peace and mind.
Life is a game; it's a game of the mind
If one plays it right, one can win the game of life…

Mind is a powerful as wind
It can keep one on his and her wings
It can blow in and out, anything
Lord Krishna gave us a hint
To conquer the world, one must conquer the mind
Life is a game; it's a game of the mind
If one plays it right, one can win the game of life…

Controlling the mind is the secret
If one wants any peace or rest
One should think and realize the true fact
That I am holy eternal spirit
Mind is only my servant.
People ignore or forget this important fact
Hence becomes victim of life
And suffers from miseries of life
Life is a game; it's the game of mind
If one plays it right, one can win the game of life…

Thoughts are product of the mind
Mind is very fertile
It produces one thought every second
These can drive one wild in no moment
One must control this process
Or else one will not have any rest
In this confusion, one can lose the game of life
Life is a game; it's a game of the mind
If one plays it right, one can win the game of life…

Emotions are another product of the mind
Emotions and intelligence are in constant conflict
One who chooses one's emotions
Has to deal with many commotions
His life can be hell
He may not get any peace or rest
One must be clear about this fact
Controlling the mind is the only tact
Or life can be a mess
Life is a game; it's a game of the mind
If one plays it right, one can win the game of life...

Mind travels faster than anything else
Its speed and rate cannot be met
Whether one wants to be at the top of the mountain,
Or the bottom of the ocean
It takes less than one second
Going to the moon, Mars or any planet
Neither has it needed any time or gadget
I wanted to compare the speed of the mind with the light
The fleeting mind made fun of the light
Light is too slow for the mind
It travels only 186,000 miles in one second
To get the speed of the mind one has to
Multiply every second
It causes dizziness and confusion
Controlling the mind is the only solution
Controlling the mind can gives one real rest
So that one can think and analyze,
Who is he? And why is he?
Life is a game; it's a game of the mind
If one plays it right, one can win the game of life...

Weak minded people have another feature
They are moody and of unpredictable nature.
They fly off the handle any second
Because their mind has no direction
They get dizzy and/or confused
And lose the game of life
Hence becomes victim of life
Life is a game; it's a game of the mind
If one plays it right one can win the game of life...

They are of weak will and determination
It is the cause of procrastination
They fear any initiation
Or leave the project without completion
It causes failure of their mission
So they get lost in the game of life,
Hence become victim of life
Life is a game; it's a game of the mind
If one plays it right, one can win the game of life…

These people have few more features
Anger, hate, jealousy worries are additional features
They cannot get rid of these creatures
Because these creatures take control of their life,
And/or become part of life
In this confusion they get lost in life
Hence suffers from pain and miseries of life
The wise gave good advice
One must get rid of these creators
If one wants any independence and freedom
This is the way to win the game of life
Life is a game; it's a game of the mind
If one plays it right, one can win the game of life…

You need to know one more secret:
The body is the product of the mind
And mind is the product of the thoughts
So by changing the thoughts, I can change the mind
By changing the mind, I could change the body
Life is a game; it's a game of the mind
If one plays it right, one can win the game of life…

Be clear and understand
That we are eternal and holy soul
Where soul is the boss and mind is only servant
Life is a continuous process
It is an eternal fact of life
One must understand oneself and this life
Who is he? And why is he?
This is the only way to win the game of life
Life is a game; it's a game of the mind
If one plays it right, one can win the game of life…

Meditation, chanting, prayer are of some help
But good word and good act is the real tact
Remember magician is the mind, and body the magic
It is the secret and fact of life
Life is a game; it's a game of the mind
If one plays it right, one can win the game of life...

No time is good and no time is bad
It is all in the present
And "present" is the "time."
Life is a game; it's a game of the mind
If one plays it, right one can win the game of life...

What is right and what is wrong?
What is good and what is bad?
It is all what you believe and what you think
Everybody is right in their own way
Life is a game; it's a game of the mind
If one plays it right one can win the game of life...

Call me Brother, Doctor, friend, Pratap or Singhal
But take my sincere advice,
You must understand and realize
That controlling the mind is the only solution
If you want to have happiness or freedom
Life is a game; it's a game of the mind
If one plays it right, one can win the game of life.

Mind

Oh my friend, make up your mind...
What can you do?
What will you do?
What can you be?
What will you be?
What should you be?
What would you be?
Make up your mind, make up.

Who is your boss?
Who is your friend?
Who is your enemy?

Who is your dear one?
Make up you mind, make up.

What should your life be?
What will your life be?
Will you behave like the dead?
Will you still be alive after death?
How should your present be?
How should your future be?
Make up your mind, make up.

What would you say?
What would you hear?
What would you see?
What would you do?
What would you eat?
What would you drink?
Make up your mind, make up.

On this planet
How long have you been here?
How long you will be here?
What have you gained?
What more will you gain?
What will be your final thought?
What will be your final word?
This is Pratap's sincere advice
If you want happiness and freedom
This is the time and the time is now
Make up your mind, make up.

CHAPTER NINETEEN

Subconscious Mind: The Final Product

What is the role of our subconscious mind in keeping us healthy and happy?

You should know that your life is the product of your habits, good and bad, because you do most things by habit. What you eat, how you dress, how you talk, what you think, and also what you do; most routine things in life is by habit.

This habit thing is known as your second nature. This second nature has its roots in the subconscious mind. So you can appreciate how the subconscious has an effect on your daily life. Okay so far?

Now understand that the most practical and useful fact is that you do have the power to break the bad habits and inculcate good habits by retraining the subconscious mind. This is the essence of this chapter!

Objectives

1. Our life is the product of our habits, good and bad.

2. All habits have their seat in the subconscious mind.

3. We do have the power to reprogram our subconscious mind.

4. We can even heal ourselves with the power of the subconscious mind (with hypnosis and meditation).

Introduction

The mind and the subconscious mind are two different entities, but they are complementary to each other. Whereas the mind is a conscious entity, the subconscious mind is not conscious. The mind has the thinking and decision-making ability, whereas the subconscious mind works like a computer databank, without thinking or reasoning ability.

Learning: a process

Learning happens in two steps. The first step in learning is analyzing, understanding, and knowing the information. The second step includes storing the information for future use. The mind and intellect play active roles in the first step, and the subconscious mind in the second step. What a team, one helping the other!

Here is an example: You decide to learn something new, like driving, cooking, math, language, art, or learning to use a computer. The mind and intellect now come into play. They struggle to comprehend, analyze, and grasp. At this stage, the subconscious mind is very passive and has no role, but once the information is learned it is stored in the subconscious mind forever. And this becomes our second nature. This second nature belongs to our subconscious mind. Now the mind and intellect are free to do anything else, like learning something new etc.

Memory

The subconscious mind is the databank. It never forgets anything. It is believed that our subconscious mind remembers each and every thing that we have ever learned either in this life (or even in the past lives). All of our habits and memories are stored in the subconscious mind. This is not true of the conscious mind, because it tends to forget. The reason people forget information is that they have not learned at the level of the subconscious mind.

This has a practical and important implication, i.e., in order to break any old habit or old learning; you need to enter into the subconscious mind to fix the past memory. This cannot be done with any medicine. Hypnosis and meditation are two modalities and/or techniques that make it easier to enter into the subconscious mind. (Hypnosis and meditation are safe, natural, and effective modalities for the treatment of many chronic physical diseases and/or mental conditions.)

Automation: a function of the subconscious mind

The subconscious mind is like autopilot or our computer. You train it once and it does the rest. No forgetting, no goofing.

Now let us see how the subconscious mind impacts our life. Swami Vivekanand has given a beautiful description of this subject in the treatise, *The Complete Works of Swami Vivekanand*:

> "We are all slaves to our sense, slaves to our own minds, conscious and subconscious. The reason why a criminal is a criminal is not because he desires to be one, but because he has not his mind under control and therefore is a slave to his own subconscious and conscious mind and to the mind of everybody else. He must follow the dominant trend of his own mind; he cannot help it. He is forced onward in spite of himself, in spite of his own better prompting, his better nature; he's forced to obey dominant mandate of his mind. The poor man cannot help himself. We see this in our own lives constantly. We are constantly doing things against the better side of our nature and afterwards we are upbraided for so doing and wonder what we could have been thinking of, how we could have done such a thing! Yet, again and again we do it, and again and again we suffer for it and upbraid ourselves. We are slaves to ourselves and to others. Deep down in our subconscious mind are stored up all the thoughts and acts of the past, not only of this life, but of all other lives we have lived. This great boundless ocean of the subconscious mind is full of all the thoughts and actions of the past. Each one us is striving to be

> recognized pushing outward for expression, surging wave after wave, out upon the objective mind the conscious mind."

So you must appreciate from the above paragraph why it is important to think, act, and do right the first time, because whatever we do shapes, programs, and prepares the subconscious mind for the subsequent acts for the remainder of life (even next lives).

Definition

The Oxford Dictionary defines the subconscious mind as that part of the mind that is not fully awake or alert, and that affects our life by the decisions and choices that we make.

The subconscious mind makes our life easier by providing automation. It is important to know that the role of the subconscious mind can be several times more potent than the conscious mind in decision-making indirectly and hence in affecting our life.

You ask why? Because most of our actions are done like a machine. What we say or do, how we drive, how we read, what we eat, and how we dress is done automatically. There are only a few things in life that require us to think. As a matter of fact some people never think, so they are like living machines; that is, they are under the total control of their subconscious mind, hence they fall into this category. I am sure you are not one of them, because you are reading this book to think and to make changes.

For interest sake it is also good to know that many authorities believe the mind has two components: the conscious and subconscious element. However, other authorities consider the subconscious mind as a separate entity and not part of the conscious mind. They label the subconscious mind as a causal body or causal element that is responsible for many deep functions of life, including birth and death cycles.

Role of the subconscious mind

In determining our future (Punishment and reward system)
According to Vedic philosophy inasmuch as our subconscious mind is our friend and a royal servant, we are also the slave of the subconscious mind. All good and bad acts or karma are coded as positive or negative, respectively. Our future will be affected/controlled by this coding. This coding, positive and negative, will affect the next day, next month, next year or subsequent lives. Now appreciate the implications of that.

- Every being is punished or rewarded by his or her positive or negative coding, and not by God. God does not deal case by case or person by person. He is too busy for this.

- Secondly, until a person cleanses their bad karma or coding, they do not get entitled to salvation or eternal happiness (Vedic view of life).

Healing with the power of the subconscious mind
I have mentioned in this chapter that our subconscious mind is the direct reflection of our thoughts, beliefs, acts, and behavior. So by changing our thoughts, belief system, and acts, we could change the subconscious mind and therefore could bring changes in our mind and/or life for the better. This is the basis of healing with hypnosis.

The subconscious mind and the super-conscious mind
The mind has three important stages in its development: the conscious mind, subconscious mind, and the super-conscious mind. The super-conscious mind is the best, ultimate, and final state of mind where one finds bliss. In order to enter the super-conscious state of mind, one has to enter the subconscious mind first.

Hypnosis and meditation are two techniques that make it easier to enter the subconscious mind. Some yogis are typical examples. They regularly enter their super-conscious mind through the subconscious mind with the power of meditation, and they then enjoy the bliss of life.

Test: Your subconscious mind

Because:

I speak the truth.	Y/N
I don't lie or steal.	Y/N
I don't have any bad habits, for example, alcohol, or drugs.	Y/N
My thoughts are usually positive and beneficial.	Y/N

As a result:

I don't have nightmares.	Y/N
I don't have any fears.	Y/N
I sleep well.	Y/N
I am at peace with myself.	Y/N
I am calm and happy by nature.	Y/N
I am funny at times.	Y/N
I can relax easily.	Y/N

If you have answered most of the questions with yes, then you have a good subconscious mind. Congratulations! Otherwise you need to work on it.

Benefits (practical aspect)

It should be clear by now that we are responsible for programming our subconscious mind. Now let us learn how to program the subconscious mind for our benefit. Good thoughts, acts, behavior, and habits have a positive and good programming effect on the subconscious mind. Conversely negative thoughts, acts, and behavior have a negative or bad programming effect on the subconscious mind. So the best, or probably the only, way to program or reprogram the subconscious mind is by the repetition of good thoughts, words, or acts. Think about it!

It is not that difficult to differentiate good thoughts, words, acts, and habits from the bad ones. We all know it well. We are told repeatedly by our teachers, parents, spiritual books, and by our conscience. In the chapter on spirituality, I have defined clearly what is good and what is bad. (See Chapter 22) The inculcation of good habits requires patience, hard work, and austerity, but it is worth the effort.

Let me give you some examples of good and bad habits. Remember these are just habits and therefore can be changed with a little patience and perseverance:

1. Some people eat healthy by nature and habit, while others eat only junk food.

2. Some people exercise regularly; others are lazy by nature.

3. Some people speak the truth; others constantly lie.

4. Some people read books and relax in their spare time; others' mind is devil's workshop.

5. Some people are always happy and content; others constantly complain.

6. Some people go to temple or church and pray; others constantly criticize God, religion or others.

7. Some people are always considerate of others; others are rude and nasty.

Can you think of some good and bad habits and make a list for better insight? The list that you make of your own habits would help you much more than the list that I have given here, because in reality your list will address your own needs or issues. It is never too late to acquire good habits. (See Chapter 1) Think about it. It is worth the time.

The key message

We need to be careful, cautious, and deliberate in every word we say, every act we perform, and every thought that comes to mind, because it also has a programming effect on the subconscious mind, and hence on our life.

Mantra **(Recite it on a daily basis for thirty days.)**

I am the product of the subconscious mind. The subconscious mind is the product of what I think, what I say, and what I do. Therefore I am careful and deliberate in what I think, what I say, and what I do.

CHAPTER TWENTY

Redefining Spiritual Health

Spiritual health is the health of the spirit, the soul, the most important part of a person. Before taking up the subject in detail, let us review the definition of spiritual health one more time. Spiritual health is part of the physical, mental, and spiritual health trio. Spiritual health determines whether one shall live the life of pain and suffering or of joy, bliss and happiness.

Spiritual Health

The hallmarks of good spiritual health are spiritual strength and stability. It has two components:

1. At the personal level: One is adept, content, and satisfied within the self. One appreciates and enjoys life.

2. At the interpersonal level: One has the feeling of oneness, so that one becomes kind and loving to all.

Examples of spiritually healthy people are:

1. Wise people
2. Spiritual masters
3. Elevated souls
4. Prophets
5. Rishi
6. Seers

The result of the spiritual health is: One is content, confident, happy, and adept.

Reverse: Let us appreciate the opposite of spiritual health:

- Impatience
- Dissatisfaction
- Complaining about people and situations
- Indifference to others

The result of the spiritual weakness is unhappiness and misery.

CHAPTER TWENTY-ONE

Soul: The Consciousness/ Awareness

O Spirit, command my soul to arise
from the sepulcher of littleness into
Thy vastness of everywhereness.
Lift its matter-caged consciousness
into omnipresent freedom in Thee.

—*Paramahansa Yogananda*

I am a soul (consciousness). You are a soul. Every living being is a soul. Soul seeks happiness. I seek happiness. You seek happiness. We all seek happiness. There is no debating about it! How one can get lost in the search of happiness is another issue. After you understand that you are a soul, hence divine and eternal, you will look at life a lot differently. Your life will begin to change for the better.

Once again coming back to the understanding of the soul, remember you are a soul. Soul equates to consciousness. The more and more you expand your consciousness, the more and more you will realize that everything is okay. Everyone is okay. All divisions are arbitrary. The past, present, and future are one. Pain and pleasures are okay. Then what and where is the problem?

Summary

The realization is that I am a soul (consciousness)→gradual expansion of consciousness to→vastness gradual homecoming of freedom and happiness.

Objectives

1. We are souls. Soul means consciousness, and consciousness is the very basis of life.

2. The vastness or expansion of consciousness (or awareness) is the cause of everlasting joy and happiness.

3. Learning to expand the consciousness or awareness (for a happy and blissful living).

Understanding the soul

The importance of the soul can be understood by the statement made by the great Swami Vivekanand, who used to say: "You can lose anything, but do not lose your soul."

Soul is consciousness. Consciousness is the greatest asset of life. An unconscious man is half dead and he may or may not recover. Super-conscious people see far and beyond. They can easily appreciate how and why everything is okay.

Consciousness varies not only from animal to man, but also from one person to another. The variation can be extreme. As you know, some people are hardly conscious or aware of what is going on at any given moment, while others can plan for the next five, ten, fifteen years or even more. When you look at the life of spiritual masters or great people, they had a plan and mission for their whole life. This is the importance of consciousness and of expanded consciousness.

Attributes
We are souls (consciousness), and the soul has two important attributes:

1. It does not die!
2. It does not suffer!

The soul does not die. (We do not die.)
It is interesting to know that most of us believe that we will not die, although we see death every day. Is it not a surprise?

Let me quote an interesting story from *Mahabharata*, one of the greatest epics of India. In *Mahabharata* there was a great religious hero whose name was Yudhistra, a king and a yogi. Once he was trapped by the king of death named Yama. He was warned that he had to die, unless he answered one of the questions of Yama. Yudhistra was asked, "What is the most wonderful surprise in this world?" He replied, "It is the persistent belief of mankind in their deathlessness. In spite of witnessing death everywhere, one continues to believe that he/she will not die." Yama was pleased with his answer and Yudhistra was set free.

In this reference, equally or probably more interesting and intriguing is this: Why it should be a surprise to anyone that we continue to believe that we will not die? Because we know in our heart that we are the soul, and the soul does not die! We have witnessed death of bodies time after time. But we (souls) are still alive. So what is the surprise if we believe in the truth that we (our soul) will not die?

The soul does not suffer.
Remember we are the souls. It is only the body and the mind that suffer. In other words we suffer only when we attach or identify ourselves with the body or the mind, but we are neither the body nor the mind. We are souls, and the soul does not suffer.

Definition of the soul

As defined by *The Oxford Dictionary*, soul is a noun. It is spiritual or non-material part of a person regarded as immortal. However, the metaphysical sciences give a better definition of the soul. It describes the soul as the only conscious entity and animating principle of life. If one is moving, eating, talking, listening, or if there is any sign of life, it is due to the soul, the consciousness. Vedas clarifies one very important fact that soul is free, and eternal. Soul is everlasting. It never dies, never takes birth.

Now one must also wonder what soul is not. It is not the mind, the intelligence, the ego, or anything else.

You all know that the word "soul" is quite abstract. I have been searching for a long time as how to best define or explain the word "soul." I have studied a lot of literature in this reference. I would like to define the soul in the following manner, because I find this definition to be universal. It can apply to the living and non-living, as well as to all issues in business and private life.

From what I understand, the soul of anything is its essence of that thing. For example, the soul of the pen is to write, and of food to nourish. If the pen doesn't write, we throw it away. If the food gets spoiled or loses its nourishing quality, we throw it away. Similarly the essence of our life is consciousness. When the soul or consciousness leaves the body, life ends, and we cremate or bury the body. Therefore, in reference to life, we could say that the soul is the consciousness, or the essence of life is consciousness.

Let us understand one more word: "spirited" which is associated with the word soul (spirit). Spirited means full of energy, enthusiasm, and determination. Spiritless means lacking courage, energy, and determination.

Let me give you a practical example of consciousness. It really defines the person. A person has at least two components to their personality:

1. The profession or the work of the person.
2. The consciousness (soul) of that person.

In every field there are different grades of people. There are different grades of doctors, nurses, engineers, accountants, attorneys, CEOs, and so on. The difference in their grade and behavior is due to the different level of their consciousness (soul), although their education level, social status, and financial background may be the similar. They may also be paid equally.

Let us say you go to the hospital. You are taken care of by a nice nurse. You feel good about it. She is caring and compassionate. She understands your needs. She looks after you. Now it is 4 p.m., and the shift changes. A new nurse takes over your case. All of a sudden you feel uncomfortable. You can't ask her for anything. You can't tell her anything. You ask for a glass of water and she forgets. Now you ask for a bedpan, but she comes two hours later. Remember both of these nurses are doing the same job. They went through the same training, and they are being paid equally. But you can appreciate the difference between these two nurses. This is due to the different conscious levels of the nurses.

This is one of the tiny examples of life. It is applicable to each and every field. It is also applicable to you and me and to everyone. Think how well we perform in our day-to-day life. Take a pause. This information is too important for you to rush!

The conscious level of a happy person is quite different from the conscious level of an average or sad person. I hope now you are clear by what I mean by consciousness or the soul of the person.

What is the seat (location) of the soul?

There are several views on this issue. Swami Omanand writes that the soul is located in the A.V. node of the heart. Other authorities believe that it is located in the medulla oblongata or pineal gland of the brain. Still others believe that the soul is located in the upper part of the body, from the heart and up.

How does the soul function?

The soul is the only conscious entity in our body. In life, nothing functions without the soul. Our body or any part of it will not function without the soul. Even the mind and intellect will not function without the soul. The soul is the animating and directing energy behind every thought, word, and act. If one is alive, they have a soul.

Cause and effect

We know that in the universe, everything is based on the cause and effect phenomenon. The subtler thing is the cause, and the grosser is the effect. Here the soul is the cause and the body is the effect, because the soul is the subtler of the two. The soul is the subject; everything else is the object. (Swami Dayanand of Saylorsburg, PA)

Expansion of consciousness: the effects of

As our consciousness expands, we see far and beyond. When we enter primary school, we learn the alphabet, and then by middle school we can read and write fluently. In high school we open our consciousness to the field of physics, chemistry, biology, arts, math, science, history, and languages. When we look at the microscope for the first time, our eyes really begin to open. With the invention of the microscope, we broadened our consciousness further and further. Now we can see with our eyes what we could not see before. Further expansion came with the invention of the electron microscope which enables us to see even the tiniest thing that was not visible even with the microscope. Not only this, but with the help of a telescope we can see far into the distance. This expansion continues with better and better inventions.

Let us look at simple day-to-day life examples. When we stand on the third or fourth floor of high-rise building, we can see much further than when we were standing on the first floor. But when we go to the tenth or eleventh floor now we can see further and further away, and when we stand on the top of the building or ninety-ninth floor, now we can see miles and miles away on a clear day. (I hope you don't have a fear of heights!) What a great feeling! It is all due to the expansion of the consciousness as we keep going up and up. Remember this is only at the physical level.

Now let us apply this expansion of consciousness at the metaphysical level. You should appreciate how people with a low level of consciousness think so differently from people with a higher level of consciousness. People with a low level of consciousness perform acts without thinking and without understanding the consequences, immediate or remote. A thief thinks that he could run away. Similarly a person who cheats thinks he will get away. But people with an average level of consciousness will not do such acts, because they know that the chances of getting caught and going to jail are high.

Now let's take the example of people with a higher level of consciousness. They can see far and beyond into the future. They know that every action brings a reaction. They know that every bad action will bring bad result sooner or later. This fact alone keeps them out of trouble. So they stay on the right path and lead a happier life.

Global vs. focal

Let me give you another example. You are looking very closely at a portrait that is ten feet by twenty feet in dimensions. You criticize the nose and eyes of one of the characters in the portrait. Suddenly somebody enters the room from the other end of the long hallway and feels awe looking at the portrait. That person is impressed with the total beauty and not just the eyes and nose of one of the subjects that you are analyzing. Suddenly you go back and stand by the person who newly arrived, and you get the same feeling. Now you are also looking at the whole portrait.

This also applies to our life. When we look at one bad day, one bad incident, or even one or two bad years of life, we forget the whole good life that we have led in the past. But when we take one incident or bad day or one bad year in context to the whole life, things look much different. This is the importance of global understanding or expansion of the consciousness.

As we continue to expand our consciousness at the metaphysical level, we learn to appreciate that nothing is that good or that bad. I am okay. You are okay. Everybody is okay. One begins to understand and accept everything and everybody as good or normal. The overview of life changes, so one does not get upset over little things. One learns to live calmly and peacefully. One begins to enjoy the life of contentment, and one begins to feel at ease and relaxed.

The practical aspect of the expansion of the consciousness can be understood by the fact that all good acts and words are a reflection of a higher level of consciousness, so are love, compassion, and kindness.

Equally true is the fact that all wrong acts, words, and deeds are a reflection of a low level of consciousness, so are lying, stealing, cheating, and fighting.

People without soul > a metaphor
There are quite a few people in this world who have no feeling, no ethics, and no principles. At times we call these people without soul (consciousness). They are totally ignorant about life. They may do things that a normal person would be ashamed to do, but they take no ill of it. They live in their own world for selfish reasons without any concern for others. They may even harm or injure others or themselves. They lack consciousness. They lack soul, speaking metaphorically.

Test

I have devised three tests. The first test is to evaluate whether the message of the chapter is clear or not; and the next two tests are for the evaluation of the self (soul). As always, these tests are for insight and not for grading and judging anyone. So please relax, enjoy, and learn.

Test # 1

I am part of the body, mind, and soul trio. Y/N

My body is the physical manifestation; my mind and soul are the metaphysical manifestation. Y/N

Every physical element in this universe must perish to be recycled again and again. Y/N

My body, being a physical element, will perish for the purpose of recycling. Y/N

My soul is my metaphysical existence and hence is eternal and forever. Y/N

The purpose of my life or the soul is to find freedom and happiness. Y/N

Freedom comes by mental and spiritual growth or by expansion of the consciousness (awareness). Y/N

In order to increase consciousness (awareness), I must be aware or conscious what I think, say, or do. Y/N

I should never do anything mechanically. Y/N

If you have answered all of the questions with yes, then you are clear about the message of this chapter. Congratulations! If not, please read this chapter again.

Test # 2

It is based upon the Vedic philosophy which states that we see ourselves in others. Applying this principle, if you believe that generally everybody is good or okay, you are also a good or okay person. However, if you believe that everybody is bad, then you should also doubt the goodness in you. This question alone should provide some insight into your own inner strengths/weaknesses. For example, a thief believes that everybody is a thief. Equally a saint believes that everyone is a saint. Similarly a gentleman believes everyone is a gentleman and treats others with respect, whereas a crook treats everyone otherwise.

Test # 3

I am not selfish. Y/N

I have no fears, anxieties, or worries. (Soul does not fear anything.) Y/N

I believe that life is an opportunity to become good and noble. Y/N

I know that life has a deep purpose which I must fulfill. Y/N

I have morals, ethics, and principles of life that I follow. Y/N

I work with my consciousness (very basic question). Y/N

I have love and compassion for others. Y/N

Result: I am a happy person. Y/N

If you have answered all or most of the questions with yes, then you are a good soul/person. This is not a test of pass or fail but for better insight and understanding.

Key message

This chapter takes one to a deepest level of being. It has two important, practical, and useful messages:

1. I am a soul and everybody is a soul. Soul means consciousness. Therefore I am eternal and forever. This should bring a sense of calmness and peace. What a great feeling!

2. Expansion of the consciousness is one of the top secrets of healthy and blissful living. The more you expand your consciousness, the more you realize that nothing is that good or that bad. Everything is okay. Everybody is okay. Everything is temporary, e.g., pain and pleasure, disease and health, ups and downs, and so on.

Practical points

Expand your consciousness or awareness: reward yourself

1. We should continuously think that we are consciousness.

2. We should think, speak, and act with consciousness, and not mechanically or reflexively.

Remember whenever we work mechanically, it is due to habit or nature, and therefore we are not using our consciousness.

3. We should understand life and its eternal nature.

4. Helping others does increase our consciousness.

5. All good words, acts, and deeds expand consciousness. In this reference Swami Vivekanad writes, whenever we do anything wicked or bad, our consciousness contracts. And whenever we do something good and positive, our consciousness expands.

6. Meditation is the fastest and easiest way of increasing awareness or consciousness.

7. Knowledge of the self and its application also greatly increases the consciousness.

Mantra **(Recite it on a daily basis for thirty days.)**

I am consciousness, and soul is my name. I am happiness, soul is my name. I am joy, soul is my name. I am the soul, the eternal.

How could I ever die, this is of great surprise

Some fear death
Others can't believe in this fact
How could I ever die?
This is of great surprise
When Yama heard these words
He got mad as hell
Yama gave the sarcastic laugh
Watch and see I'll kill you all
Yama has no mercy, because that is his job
He is the king of the death, and the dead

But when Yama saw the soul
He became pale and stunned
Now it is time to lose or run
People rob, steal, and cheat to get rich and hefty
Wise tells us, don't kill the soul, for little wealth
It will be burden and sin, for which you may
have to repent.

Are you the soul, the body, or both?
If you are the body you have to die
If you believe in the soul, then you are for eternity
What do you know, and what do you believe
It matters in the end.

If I believe I am the soul
How could I ever die?
This is of great surprise!!

Behold what Pratap has to say
Always remember you are a soul
Then how could you die
This could be the best surprise!

CHAPTER TWENTY-TWO

Spirituality: Path of Freedom & Happiness

Spirituality breeds happiness. Spirituality means oneness: with the self, with each other, and with God, where everybody and everything is okay. This is spirituality.

To reach the right destination, we need to follow the right path. Since we are spirit, spirituality is our right path. Spirituality is not only the path of oneness, but also the path of higher self (vs. lower self). It is the path of divinity, joy, freedom, and happiness vs. that of misery, pain, suffering, and dependency.

Vedas (the book of knowledge) states: "Oh, man, you are divine and make others divine." This is spirituality: The word divine has a special meaning. Let us define and understand the word divine. *The Oxford Dictionary* defines the word divine as supernatural, with magical insight into the future. The French word *diviner* means to predict. The word divine also means sacred, godly, excellent, and superb.

There are all kinds of people in this world. Some are always upbeat, smiling, and pleasant to deal with and ready to help. They are calm and content. The most important element that I have noticed in these people is that they have patience and are kind-hearted. They care for others. They may go out of their way to help others. These are spiritual people. These people are very special. Do you recall ever meeting these people in your life?

On the contrary, some people are always searching for more and more for themselves. They are impatient and restless. They are always in a rush. They are selfish and miserable. Selfishness and misery are very much related and/or connected. Selfishness and spirituality are two opposite paths. Selfishness provides materialism, wealth, and attachment, but at the cost of happiness. The ignorant and the naïve choose the path of selfishness and materialism, because it looks attractive: whereas spirituality is the path of altruism, higher self and lasting happiness. Only the awakened soul chooses this path.

Objectives

1. We must remember that we are spirits and spirituality is our path.
2. Spirituality is the path of oneness.
3. The spiritual path is the path of joy, freedom, and happiness.

Introduction

You know that in life we do two things:

1. Help oneself (a common denominator of all living creatures, including animals)
2. Help others (more applicable to human beings and especially to spiritual people)

Any doubt about it? Nope!

Helping ourselves is a natural and innate quality of every living being from the tiniest bacteria to the largest elephant, and human beings are no exception to this principle of life. Helping one another is the basis of the human life. Helping one another bonds us or keeps us together, whether it is among family members, social circles or in the business world.

When you go to any business place, the first thing you hear is, "May I help you?" Is it not true?

Now appreciate how helping is related to spirituality: Spirituality takes us one step further. The more sincerely, more compassionately, more lovingly, more selflessly, and more dedicatedly we help others, the more spiritual we become. Think about it! Take a break! Meditate on this thought! This has been the quality of all the great people of this planet. It is also one of the ways to rise spiritually.

The personality of the spiritual people

Spiritual people are pleasant and have the ability to influence others. They have patience and a deep sense of contentment. They have a feeling of blessedness. They can adapt to different situations and circumstances. They have faith in self and in the supreme, and therefore they have no fears, worries, or anxieties. They have love and compassion for all; they enjoy a feeling of oneness.

Definition

Spirituality means the doctrine, the spirit that exists as distinct from the matter or the body. Spirituality is related to the soul or spirit. Spirituality is the path of higher self.

Religion vs. spirituality

Religion and spirituality are quite different. The differences must be understood clearly. Spirituality is a universal phenomenon and does not relate to religion, caste, or sex, whereas religion is a confined word that describes faith of certain people or even locality.

Materialism vs. spirituality

Materialism is related to selfishness, attachment, dependency, and thus loss of freedom, whereas spirituality is related to oneness and freedom. These are two different paths. Let us appreciate and analyze the differences:

M- Materialism S- Spirituality

M: What is in it for me (without being considerate of others)?
S: What is in it for everybody?

M: Needs of your body
S: Needs of your eternal soul (happiness and bliss)

M: Bonding and attachments to mundane things
S: Bonding with spiritual elements

M: Taking it in and growing physically
S: Giving, sharing out of love and kindness, and growing spiritually

M: Growing by hook and by crook
S: Growing only by fair and just means

M: Shortsightedness
S: Insight and foresight

M: Short term gain
S: The ultimate gain, the long term gain

M: Talking and being dogmatic
S: Listening, thinking, and understanding

M: Complaining about people
S: Listening and helping people

M: Revenge and getting stuck
S: Forgiveness and moving ahead

M: Focal understanding only with one's own perspective
S: Global understanding

M: Advising and criticize others
S: Helping others

M: Non-acceptance of self and others, or acceptance of self only
S: Acceptance of self and all others (everybody is okay)

M: Lack of faith in self and in the supreme, thus full of anxieties and fears
S: Faith in self and in the supreme, therefore no anxiety, no worries, rather patience and calmness

M. Action, hustle and bustle
S. Restful, calm and at peace

What is the opposite of spirituality?

Although I have tried to describe the path of spirituality in the best possible way, sometimes the subject matter becomes clearer when we can understand the opposite of it. You must remember that whatever weakens the mind and spirit is against the path of spirituality. Now let us try to understand what could be the opposite of spirituality:

Personal level
- The ignorant fact that I am the body
- Selfishness, irrespective of how it affects others
- Materialism (unfair means)

Interpersonal level
- Indifference to the feelings of others
- Thinking, speaking, or doing bad
- Not caring for others
- Lack of love and kindness for others

Spiritual people: Real life examples

You will notice in the following examples that education, social status, and financial background has very little to do with spirituality.

Spirituality of a laborer (narrated by Achara Vajeesh Ji)

Everywhere there are good and bad people, rich and poor, materialistic and spiritual, mean and divine. Here is the story of a small town where a temple was being built.

As the temple was being constructed, there were three laborers working side by side. A big sign read TEMPLE UNDER CONSTRUCTION.

A great swami was visiting that place. He asked one of the laborers "What are you doing?" He replied angrily "Can't you read? You are an intelligent person and not like me. A temple is being built. We have to feed our stomachs; we have to work in the heat and cold."

That great swami now asked the second laborer, "What are you doing?" He replied: "Sir, here the temple is under construction, and I am just doing my job. The rest I do not know."

Now the great swami asked the third laborer, "What are you doing?" He states "Oh, great man, listen, a temple is being constructed here. People will come to pray and will get the blessings of God. They will find comfort in their soul and heart. I am overjoyed with this feeling, because I am part of this holy project."

From the above story, we can appreciate the feelings of the three laborers. All the three laborers were doing the same job, but each one perceived their work differently. You can imagine how the perception of the same work would affect the life in a different manner. To the first laborer, the temple work is a load. To the second laborer, the temple work is just like any other building. To the last laborer, it is an honor and joy to be part of such a project.

The lesson

Now for a moment take a break. Look at your life and work. How do you take your work? Question yourself. Let today be the opportunity to take stock of your life! Remember spirituality does not live or reside in temples or churches, but in the heart and soul of each human being.

The spiritual master: a meeting experience

Have you ever met a spiritual person? What pleasant feeling of ease and comfort do they impart? Fortunately I have had several experiences of meeting spiritual people in my life. What a joy, what a feeling of calmness, sense of contentment, and peace!

You feel at ease in their company, and their words are comforting. They are so content that you also begin to feel content. They are at peace, and you also begin to feel at peace. The feeling when you meet them is similar to the feeling when you go to a temple or place of sanctity. They make you feel important. They care for you because they are kind-hearted. They are not in a rush. They have patience because to them you are an important soul.

Good and bad: Differentiation

Is there really a test which could differentiate good from bad? Before I answer that question let me make two statements in this reference. Number one: differentiation from good and bad may not always be easy, and number two we are not supposed to judge anyone. However if we are doing so, without any malice and solely for the sake of self-improvement, I believe it should be okay.

I have devised these tests based on the Vedic system. Vedas (the book of knowledge) states that I am "three in one, i.e., I am the observer, I am the observation, I am being observed." In nutshell it means that we see others as we are. Let us see how this can be applied to our daily practical life.

Test # 1: Role reversal

It is easy to understand once you learn and play the game of role reversal. For example, if you think, say or do something to others, think how you would feel if you were in their shoes. (In other words, exchange places with the other person.) If doing so it would make you feel bad, then your actions are bad, and if it would make you feel good, then your actions are good.

Test # 2

Anything that will benefit all, including you, will be good; anything that can be harmful to anyone, including you, will be bad.

Test # 3

Whatever thought, word, or action we like to keep secret or hidden is usually bad. Conversely whatever thought, word, or action we like to share or tell others is usually a sign of goodness.

Test # 4

If you believe that people either are good or okay, then you are also good and okay. If you believe 50 percent of the people are good, then you are only 50 percent good. If you believe that only 20 percent of people are good, then your goodness is only at the 20 percent level, and so on.

Test # 5

A person who looks for good in others is usually a good person. Conversely, a person who is always looking for what is bad in others cannot be a good person.

Test # 6

This is a simpler test. "A good person is one who thinks, says, and does good things."

Evaluation

Am I a spiritual person?

The importance of this test is to understand whether or not you are on the path of spirituality, which is the path of higher self, oneness, and also of happiness.

<u>Personal level</u>

I understand that I am spirit and not this body.	Y/N
I understand that life has a deep purpose; it is not just to eat, drink, and have fun.	Y/N
I understand that I should work with my consciousness.	Y/N
I am content and at peace with myself.	Y/N
I love to read and admire the life of great people, saints, rishis, gurus or spiritual masters.	Y/N
I have no fears.	Y/N
I am a confident person.	Y/N

<u>Interpersonal level</u>

Everybody is a special person like me.	Y/N
I believe we are all created equal.	Y/N
I understand the universal principle, "As you sow, so shall you reap?"	Y/N

I have compassion and love for all.	Y/N
I feel pain when I see others in pain and suffering.	Y/N
I feel joy when I see joy in others.	Y/N
I believe everybody is okay.	Y/N
I avoid arguments.	Y/N
I avoid criticism of others.	Y/N
I don't take advantage of others.	Y/N
I try not to change or convert others.	Y/N

If you have answered most or all the questions with yes, then you are a spiritual person. If you did not pass the test, it is time for insight. Please read this chapter again or meditate.

Benefits of a spiritual path

Spirituality is the path of higher self, divinity, oneness, and inner joy. It brings us closer to each other as one big human family. It has the following implications:

1. It removes all fears.
2. It brings us all closer to each other.
3. It creates love and compassion.
4. It opens the heart (or broadens one's outlook towards others).
5. It strengthens the soul. The strengthening of the soul means joy and happiness.

The path of spirituality: outline and practice

Since the path of spirituality is so good, let us learn how we can adapt this path to our life in a simple and practical manner. To recapitulate, the path of spirituality has two components:

Personal level and interpersonal level

Personal level
One can become spiritual by becoming good, noble, and excellent.

Interpersonal level
One can become spiritual by following one or all of the three practical steps:

a. Concept of oneness: Feeling and believing
b. Universal prayer (to follow): Practicing the message
c. Spiritual phrases: Practicing the message

Now let us explore these three points.

Concept of oneness
We are all part of one big human family in which everyone is either a brother or a sister. Oneness can also be translated into four practical words:

1. Truth
2. Kindness
3. Love
4. Patience

The Universal Prayer (from Vedas)
The Sanskrit version first, followed by the English translation

Sarvay bhavantu sukhinah
Sarvay santu niraamayaah,
Sarvay bhadraani pashyantu
Maa kashchid dhukka bhaaga bhavayt.

The English translation of the prayer:
May one and all be happy and in comfort!
May one and all be happy and in good health!
May one and all do well and be happy!
May one and all be blissfully free,
from anxiety, want, and suffering!

Behold the meaning and the depth of the universal or spiritual prayer from Vedas.

The spiritual phrases

1. May I help you?
2. Can I do anything else for you?
3. I understand your pain and feeling.
4. I would not harm or hurt you or anyone!
5. I know you are a special person like everyone else.
6. I show pleasure and happiness when meeting anyone.

These are the extracts of the path of spirituality. I believe if we can practice these from the heart and soul, we will travel on the path of spirituality. We will find joy and happiness. Our consciousness and awareness will expand. We can liberate ourselves from pettiness and enter into the vastness of the universe, where everything is joy and bliss.

The key message

Just say a few kind words from your heart and soul and not just from your mouth on a daily basis. See your life sparkle and change, as well as that of others. Think about it!

If you walk on this Earth and under the sun, "with the desire, intent, and willingness to help others," you will become spiritual, and this is spirituality.

Mantra (Recite it on a daily basis for thirty days.)

I walk on this Earth and under the sun with love, kindness, and compassion for all human beings, because I am a spiritual person. I am spirit. Spirituality is my path.

My friend, it is a secret of life…

Some don’t know how to live
Some don’t know how to die
Some are dead while still alive
Others are still alive after death
Alive still are Jesus, Rama, Krishna,
Dayanand, Mohammad and many many more
But we forgot who died the week before
Because they did not know how to live or die.
My friend, it is a secret of life.

When somebody knocks at the door,
Some wonder who is here to bother
Or an opportunity to help and cater
Some love to share what they have
For others it is a burden, loss or and nuisance.
Few kind and loving words
When coming from the heart and soul
Can sparkle and change yours and others life
My friend, it is a secret of life.

When one wins a game, one feels happy and proud
But when I pretend to lose to the little one
The joy with which the little twinkles is more fun
It is confusing when to lose and when to win
Winning and losing is the game of its own kind
My friend, it is a secret of life.

Some kill or die, to win
For others peace is more important than to win
The best game is to win and let other win
Win and win is the advice of the wise
My friend, it is a secret of life.

Some can harm and injure
And can do anything for the revenge
Behold what Jesus said,
Oh my lord! Forgive the ignorant one
These are innocent in your world.
He knew only how to be kind
My friend, it is a secret of life.

There was a guru, bhakat, and yogi
People called him Dayanand Swami
Who was poisoned by his cook,
for little wealth and what else.
Jaganath was the name of the cook
Just before the death,
Said Dayanand, oh Jaganath run and run
They kill you, the way you kill me
I have come only to save, and not to kill
It was him, and it was only him
He was loving and kind
My friend, it is a secret of life.

It is the story of Lord Krishna and Sudama
Once they got stranded in a jungle
In the scary dark and the heavy rain
They were little kids, what did they know
Sudama ate the share of the Krishna
He could not resist his hunger and the rice
Sudama mother when knew of the act,
She got mad and yelled, oh Sudama
You bought poverty in your heart,
Later on it became real fact
How the little one could know,
What is wrong and what is right
My friend, it is a secret of life

Some give a dollar
And spend ten to let others know
Others give one, to get back two
I tell you a story of a king who gave day and night
Somebody asked, Oh dear king
Are you not proud and fortunate?
The king replied neither it is me, nor it is mine
It all belong to the Lord, and I belong to thee
It is He who owns us all
I am just following his command
He was humble and wise
My friend, it is a secret of life.

You call me friend, Brother Singhal or Pratap
Or Mahasha if you please

But take my heartfelt advice
Nobody wins and nobody loses
In the end everybody is even
You can check out at the end of the day, month, or life
My friend, it is a secret of life.

SECTION III

Methods & Means for a Happier Life

You must have come to the realization by now that the pursuit of good health and happiness is not a one-time deal, but an ongoing process. The moment you slack off, you can end up back at Square One. All the chapters in this section will prepare you to achieve and maintain that goal on an ongoing basis, so that you can always be victorious in your mission and in your life.

CHAPTER TWENTY-THREE

Sleep, Rest & Relaxation

Sleep, rest, and relaxation make the body, mind, and the spirit livelier, so that we can think clearly, work hard, and enjoy life.

As sleep charges the body, rest and relaxation are essential to charge the mind, and peaceful time is essential for introspection and reflection on life for the spirit. However, there is a documented story of a yogi who never used to sleep, and another story of a yogi who never ate after a certain incident in her life. (These stories are narrated and documented in the book *Autobiography of Yogi* written by: Swami Yogananda Parmahansa.)

Objectives

As sleep is essential for the body, so are rest, relaxation, enjoyment, and peaceful time for the mind and spirit.

It is easy to get rest and a good night sleep with little training

Sleep

Introduction

<u>Restorative mechanism</u>

We can easily appreciate the importance of sleep in the revival of the body's energy. When we have been working too hard or have exhausted all of our energy, the first thing that comes to our mind is sleep and long sleep. And when we wake up, the first words that we often utter are: I feel like a million. Such is the magic of sleep.

Sleep and food are two common mechanisms for replenishing the depleted energy of the body. Healthy and refreshing sleep is a gift that we can own with little practice. After sleep, we become calm; intellect is revived; and the body is refreshed. We may be ready to take on the world.

If we really want to appreciate the importance of sleep, look at the face of a sleep-deprived people, for example, soldiers coming from war; or a police officer after an all-night call; or exhausted doctors coming from duty; or a trial attorney who has been working on a tough case.

Definition of sleep

The dictionary defines sleep as: "the natural and periodic suspension of consciousness, during which bodily powers are restored."

Purpose of sleep

1. It refreshes the body and mind.
2. It is the time for repair of the day's wear and tear.
3. It makes one forget trivial annoyances of the previous day and also prepares for the next day.
4. It improves the clarity of the thought process.
5. It brings new hope and rejuvenation.

Time and sleep relationship

Time to sleep

"Early to bed early to rise makes a man healthy, wealthy, and wise." It is a good ancient phrase and worthy of our attention. The best time to sleep is from 10 p.m. to 5 a.m., according to Ayurveda (science of life). A little variation is okay, as long as there is regularity in the sleeping schedule. That means one should try to keep fixed sleep schedule (a big plus).

Time spent in sleep in a lifetime

Sleep constitutes at least 25 to 33 percent of our lifetime. To some people, it may be 40 to 50 percent of their lifetime (a little too much). Excessive sleep does waste time. If you sleep 6 hours a day (one-fourth of the day), it will amount to 3 months in a year. But if you sleep 8 hours a day (one-third of a day), it will amount to 4 months in a year. However, some people sleep 12 hours a day (half a day), which means 6 months in a year.

Now think, how old are you? How much time have you spent sleeping? You can calculate easily from the above formula. For example, if you sleep 6 months a year, and you are 50 years old that means you have spent 25years in sleep. But if you sleep only 4 months a year, you have spent 16½ years in sleep.

A true story: In one of the epics of India, there was a person known as Kumbhkaran (brother of King Ravana). He used to sleep 12 hours a day and was also a glutton. In India, people call a person a Kumbhkaran who sleeps 12 hours a day. Some people have misinterpreted that Kumbhkaran used to sleep 6 months on and 6 months off. However, this is not the case.

Years you have slept: the formula

Time spent in sleep in your life = your age in years ÷ (24 ÷ hours you sleep each night) For example, you are 30 years old, and you sleep 8 hours a night. Now apply the formula: 30 years ÷ (24 ÷ 8 hours) = 10 years.

How many hours should you sleep?

It can vary from person to person. You can sleep as little or as much as you need to feel refreshed. It is important that you feel refreshed after sleep. If you require 12 hours of sleep, it is okay, but you should think how much time is being spent in sleep (6 months in a year).

On average, people sleep between 6 to 8 hours. Small children, babies, teenagers, medical students on vacation, and medical residents coming off call after a heavy night's schedule may need more time to sleep for recuperation. Military personnel after war need extra sleep. Also college students coming home during the summer may sleep twelve hours a night. That is a recovery or recuperation period and cannot be considered a regular sleep pattern.

How to reduce sleep time

Many people feel they sleep too much and wish to cut down on their sleep time. There are several ways to do that. It is easy, but one must make up their mind first. Following are some of the points which can provide help:

1. Don't eat two to three hours before going to bed.

2. Do not eat anything sweet or heavy at night; rather eat salty foods or a light evening dinner.

3. Just before going to bed, pray for two minutes or reflect on the thought that you will wake up at such and such time, for example, 4 a.m. or 5 a.m. Meditate on this point. This will help you to wake up as per your determination.

The regulation of sleep is still the single most important factor. It will be discussed later in this chapter.

Sleep and related matters

Sleep Positions

You should try to sleep on your side, either the right or the left, as it suits you. Do not sleep on your stomach. It is also not good to sleep on your back for long. However sleeping on your back for a brief period of time may be okay and relaxing, but sleeping overnight on your back without a pillow under your knees can cause back problems.

Dreams

Almost everybody dreams at night, although most people do not remember their dreams, because they do not pay attention to their dreams (as most people do not pay attention to a lot of activities of life). The best sleep is without a dream which has a special name in Ayurveda. Dreams are okay as long as they are not disturbing and/or bothersome. Sleep, disturbed by dreams, is a sign of mental tension.

Sleeping with a partner or child

Sleeping with somebody is typically a part of western culture. It is not recommended, according to Vedas. You should not be offended by this statement, because I am saying as Vedas teaches us. This is for insight only. You can make your own decision. You do not have to agree with me on this. You can do your own experiment. But you can easily appreciate that when you sleep with somebody, it not only disturbs your partner, but also your partner disturbs you whenever they change positions, toss and turn, or get up to go to the bathroom. Sleeping in the same room in two different beds is probably better than sleeping together for the couple, at least in later years of life.

Snoring

People who snore a lot may benefit greatly if they sleep on either side and avoid sleeping on their back. Although I do not recommend sleeping on the stomach, people who snore may benefit if they sleep on their side or on their stomach.

Relaxation or rest before a meal

Have you ever tried resting or even sleeping for ten to fifteen minutes before the main meal of the day? It is especially good for people who have a poor appetite. It can help your digestion and help you relax. But do not sleep immediately after any meal, especially a heavy meal. You may sleep two hours after a meal.

Why do some people have sleep problems?

There are many reasons, including:

- Irregular sleeping habits – probably one of the major causes. Learn from the people who have good sleeping habits; they have a fixed sleep schedule.
- Hunger at the time of going to bed
- Exercising late at night which stimulates one's system
- Use of stimulants, such as spicy foods, tea, coffee, and so on
- Daytime dozing
- Anxieties and worries. (It is a very important cause)
- Depression
- Hyperactivity of the mind – watching exciting shows or reading exciting books or being under bright lights especially during late evening hours

Mind and the soul: also need rest

We all need to charge ourselves at regular intervals. As sleep is one of the charging mechanisms for the body; similarly rest, relaxation, peace, silence, and meditation are important for the mind and the spirit. Rest to the mind and spirit are at least as important as, if not more than, the body for health and well being. People who are workaholics or are materialistic or spend too much time in activities suffer from mental tension, high blood pressure, and physical diseases. They are relatively tenser, less mentally stable, and unhappier than those whose life is better balanced and who find time for rest, relaxation, peace, silence, meditation, and/or prayer. (Silence, meditation, and prayer are discussed in different chapters of this book.)

Get a good night's sleep and feel like a million

Healthy, refreshing sleep is a symbol of a healthy body and mind. People who are mentally and physically healthy also sleep better. We all know the value of a good night's sleep. The important fact is that we all can enjoy refreshing sleep if we follow certain guidelines. I can summarize the important ones in few lines as follows:

<u>General</u>

- Regulate your sleep schedule: the more regular the sleep schedule, the less likely you will have sleep problems.

- Early to bed or early to rise does make one sleep better.

- Use of the alarm is an excellent idea, but do not use the snooze button. The best thing is to get up either when the alarm goes off or a minute before that. Getting up one minute before the alarm goes off can also build will power and improve sleep.

- Associate bed with sleep only and not for any other activity. For example, reading, watching TV, and socializing should not be done in bed.

Physical

- Don't eat heavy foods late at night.

- Don't drink liquids late at night; otherwise you have to get up to urinate.

- Don't exercise late at night.

- Avoid stimulants at night, e.g., coffee, tea.

Mental

- Do relaxing activities thirty minutes before you go to bed, for example, read a religious book or meditate, pray.

- Get rid of anxieties and worries. (Leave them to someone else or maybe put them in a locker for the night.)

- Think positive and good thoughts to make you calmer and more relaxed and thus sleep better.

Prescription

- Eat a half ounce of raisins before going to bed.

- Drink milk and honey at night or take toast and honey, if milk is not suitable for you.

- Try to sleep in a north and south direction for the magnetic effect.

- Listen to soothing music before going to bed (even with headphones only if needing extra help).

- Have a fixed schedule of sleep which is more effective than any other element alone.

Arise and awake!

Arise and awake has much deeper connotation than just rising from sleep. People can be sleep physically, mentally or spiritually. Physical sleep is healthy when it is in balance with the wakeup period, but the mental and spiritual sleep can be disastrous.

Sometimes we say to our friends or dear ones, wake up! See what is going on around you. Do something. This has a deeper meaning. These words relate to the spirit and the mind, and not to the sleep.

The key message

Sleep, rest, and relaxation are essential and complementary ingredients of life, so that one can stay alert, work hard, and enjoy life.

Mantra

The way I provide rest to my body, I shall also provide rest and relaxation for my mind and soul for a better healthier, longer, and happier life. I shall enjoy a good night's sleep from now on because it is all under my control.

Poem: Wake up

Wake up my friend!
Wake up!
How long will you sleep
How much will you sleep?
Wake up, my friend
Wake up!

When you sleep your work suffers
When you work your sleep suffers
Should not they compromise?
Whose side will you take?
Wake up, my friend
Wake up!

Sometimes work does not let you sleep
Sometimes sleep don't let you work
Wake up, my friend
Wake up!

Excess of anything is bad
That applies to work and sleep
Wake up, my friend
Wake up!

Wake up physically from the bed!
Mentally from the illusion and delusions
Spiritually from the darkness
Wake up, my friend
Wake up!

CHAPTER TWENTY-FOUR

Exercises for Body, Mind & Soul (Spirit)

The one way to make our body, mind, and spirit stronger is to exercise these elements. Do you agree with me on this? Exercise also is probably the best modality by which one can:

- Increase one's energy level
- Increase one's balance
- Maintain/sustain one's present limit or capacity
- Increase one's present limit or capacity
- Increase metabolism

Since we exist at three levels, we need to exercise all the levels. In this chapter I shall discuss exercises for the body, mind, and spirit.

Jack LaLanne, a ninety-year-old man, the founder of a health spa, is in excellent shape. He was asked "Do you like to exercise?" He replied, "I hate exercising, every bit of it. But I still do it because I love to be healthy."

I agree with his statement, because I also hate exercising. I bet I hate it more than he does. But I also do exercise because it makes me feel better. Probably this is true of most people.

We remember during school days, how students are given physical drills, math exercises, English exercises, writing exercises, speaking exercises, drama rehearsals, and so on, some of which are physical, others mental. The chief goal of these exercises is to prepare for the best or the worst.

Most organizations also have devised different exercise/drill programs with a similar goal in mind. They have named it in their own terms, for example, fire drill, disaster drill, emergency drill, military drill, blackout drill, and so on.

Objectives

- Exercise is one of the most essential elements for the prevention of disease and maintenance of good health.
- Exercise is also the key element for improving and extending beyond one's present limitation/capacity and for gaining strength.
- Exercise can be tailored according to the needs of each and every one, including the sick, disabled, and bedridden.
- We do need to exercise not just the body, but also the mind and the soul for better health.

Introduction

Exercise is one of our best friends. Exercise prepares us for the best and the worst of situations in life. It provides the opportunity for us to become better and stronger. We need to exercise each and every muscle, each and every faculty of the body, mind, and soul. Exercise is important not only for disease prevention, health maintenance and prevention of atrophy, but also for increasing endurance, building stamina, and building flexibility.

Keeping fit physically, mentally, and spiritually makes us not only healthy and happy but it also builds confidence and makes life easier. The time spent in exercising can be considered as one of the best investments for a healthier, longer, and happier life. Exercise makes a weak person stronger; a rigid and stiff person more flexible; and a person who can barely walk start to run. A fat person can become thin. A frail and weakly person can become stronger, and so on.

The training of the brain also helps; as a result, an uneducated person becomes educated. Mental exercises can help a person with an unstable mind to become mentally more stable. Of course there are spiritual exercises which can convert inhuman beings, into human beings.

Definition

According to the dictionary, exercise is “physical activity carried out for the sake of health and fitness. An activity carried out for a specific purpose or the application of a faculty” or “a task done to develop a skill.” Probably this is a better and broader definition as it covers mental and spiritual exercises as well.

Why some people don’t exercise: misconceptions and myths

- Takes too much time
- Requires a lot of equipment
- Fear of falling
- Upbringing; in many families exercise has no place.
- Laziness
- Belief that exercising is not for everybody; it is for athletes, runner, or school students.

Let me answer these misconceptions and myths in a few words. You do not need much time to exercise. You do not need special equipment. You do not need to join an expensive health spa. Your fear of falling will disappear soon as you start an exercise program. Exercise is a necessity for each and everyone.

Duration of exercise

This varies from individual to individual, and also on the goal one has in his or her mind. If one is an athlete preparing for the Olympics, a lot of intense exercise may be required. Dr. Laurence Morehouse, PhD and Leonard Gross in their book, *Total Fitness in 30 Minutes a Week,* have suggested as little as ten minutes at a time three days a week for an exercise program. However, this book is quite old.

I personally believe that we need to exercise on a daily basis, especially yoga. Dr. Linda Page has recommended even one-minute exercises for people who have a very busy schedule, in lieu of no exercise. However, modern authorities recommend thirty minutes of exercise three times a week for a total of ninety minutes. The benefits of the exercise are cumulative.

The intensity of exercise is also important to raise the heart rate to the target rate. The formula is: 220 minus your age and multiplied by 8/10 or (80 percent). This calculation gives your target heart rate. Let's say you are 50 years old; now apply this example: 220 minus 50 = 170 times 8/10 = 136. That is your target heart rate. In other words you must reach your target heart rate during exercise.

The effects of exercise on health, positive and negative

Although exercise has multiple benefits, if done in excess and for prolonged periods of time, it may also have some negative impact on your body. Let us first understand the benefits of exercise.

The benefits of exercise

Exercise has benefits at all levels, i.e., physical, mental, and spiritual. It keeps one young and retards the aging process.

Exercise also lowers the incidence of heart attacks, diabetes mellitus, high blood pressure, stroke, osteoporosis, and a host of other diseases.

Exercise benefits are dose-dependent to a degree. Moderate exercise is the best. However, even mild exercise has great benefits.

Some negative aspects of exercise

Strenuous exercise may have certain disadvantages, especially when carried out over a long period of time. However, the benefits of mild to moderate exercising far outweigh the risks and disadvantages. Nothing in life is 100 percent good or 100 percent bad. It does take time; it does wear down certain parts or joints due to overuse (especially heavy exercises). For example, runners have problems with their knees; boxers have problems with their brain. Swimmers often have problems with their shoulders, and so on. On rare occasions, people have collapsed, passed out, or even died during exercise. However, this should not deter one from exercising. You must consult your physician before starting a heavy exercise program.

"Exercise deficiency"

According to Prophet Edgar Cayce, "exercise deficiency" is a disease in itself and has multiple disadvantages.

Physical exercises

The manner and method used for exercising the body are multiple and varied. All have their own benefits and qualifications. The following may not be the complete list of exercise types, but it is a fairly good list.

- Aerobic
- Calisthenics (sit-ups, push-ups, jumping jacks, gymnastics)
- Isometric (weight lifting)
- Walking (forward and backward)

- Stretching exercises

- Mini trampoline exercises. Dr. Harvey and Marilyn Diamond in their book, *Fit for Life II*, discuss this extensively. They have devoted several pages to the advantages and techniques of the trampoline exercises. These are demonstrated by graphics and are easy to understand and follow.

- Rope jumping

- Resistance exercises (very good especially in later years)

- Yoga exercises have the following benefits:

    - Improving coordination of respiration, body, and mind

    - Strengthening the back

    - Increasing the flexibility of the back and the joints of the body (yoga exercise do not increase the endurance)

    - Calming the mind (Balances the mind)

    - Prolonging life

    - Uniquely, involving each and every part of the body, not just the muscles and the bones, e.g., also to include exercises for the eyes, ears, nose, throat, stomach, heart, lungs, etc. This is one of the important differentiating features from the regular exercise program. Regular exercise programs focus only on the muscle and the joints, and not any internal organs of the body.

<u>Abdominal exercises (yoga)</u>

Abdominal exercises are some of the best yogic exercises for improving digestion, improving breathing, increasing oxygenation, and stimulating the parasympathetic nervous system (for calming the mind). It is well known that the worst place for fat deposits is the abdomen, not the buttocks. Fat deposited in the abdomen interferes not only with the breathing but also with the digestive process.

Internal exercises (Taoism)

Internal exercises are those for the internal organs of the body, e.g., the eyes, ears, nose, throat, heart, lungs, abdomen, and so on. Exercises of the internal organs are also an integral part of the yogic exercise program. Internal exercises are demonstrated beautifully by Dr. Stephen Chang in his book, *The Complete System of Self Healing: Internal Exercises*. The basic principle of these exercises is that you do not need to exert much effort physically, but there is much imagination (or mental imagery) in addition to some stretching. Internal exercises, like the yogic exercises, build confidence and strengthen the mind. These exercises do not build endurance, as with yogic exercises.

One-minute exercises

Dr. Linda Page discusses the "one-minute exercise" program in her book, *Healthy Healing*. It is a good exercise program if you are short of time. For details please refer to her book.

Please remember that the benefits of exercise can be greatly increased by keeping the mind focused on the part of the body being exercised.

Mental and spiritual exercises

So far, I have been discussing physical exercises. It should be clear to you that we can and should exercise the mind and the spirit, as well. Exercising the mind makes one stable, and exercising the spirit makes one calm and content within the self. For a detailed description of mental and spiritual exercises, refer to the chapter on yoga (Chapter 29) and to the chapter on happiness (Chapter 30). But I shall state in brief some exercises here.

Mental exercises

1. Learning and practicing to stay calm and balanced in all situations, negative as well as positive.

2. Learning to understand what can or cannot be changed. You should make every attempt to change what is under your control, but also to accept what cannot be changed. This is half the battle.

3. Learning to increase concentration, observe silence, meditate, and relax.

4. Inculcating thoughts that are true, beneficial, and positive. (Such thoughts can be found in scriptures, healing affirmations, and positive affirmation.)

Spiritual exercises

The real nature of the person is the soul or the eternal spirit. Here are some spiritual exercises:

Personal level

- Understanding that life is continuum (eternal), we do not die

- Understanding that we are complete and whole, and therefore free and independent

- Trying to stay content and at peace within self

- Trying to get rid of the ego for a relaxed life

Interpersonal level

One should inculcate the feelings of love, kindness, and compassion for all. The feeling of oneness also needs to be inculcated, because it is only then that one becomes part of the one universal energy.

Practical points

A. Lack of exercise or "exercise deficiency" is a cause of multiple diseases at the physical, mental, and spiritual levels.

B. We all must have an exercise program tailored to our needs. It is easy, because there is so much to choose from.

C. We can sincerely appreciate the benefits of exercising only, after we start to exercise. So:

- Start exercising today and now.
- Although certain duration and the amount of exercise are recommended for the maximum benefits, any exercise is far better than no exercise.
- Start slow and build gradually.
- Get involved 100 percent with the body and mind. Focus the mind on the part being exercised
- Begin to experience and feel that:

  1. You are getting younger.
  2. You are becoming toned up.
  3. You are becoming healthier.
  4. You are getting rid of the toxins.
  5. You are seeing the shine on your face.
  6. You appreciate the surge of energy.

Remember that to get a good result in any field, you need to make a commitment.

The key message

Please exercise, exercise, and exercise. Any exercise is better than no exercise.

- Exercise the body.
- Exercise the mind.
- Exercise the soul.

Mantra

Exercise is extremely important for my health and well being. Since I exist at three levels—physical, mental, and spiritual—I shall exercise all the three elements, as I have learned in this chapter.

CHAPTER TWENTY-FIVE

Food & Nourishment (Part I)

Every living entity needs energy in the form of food or nourishment, including us. Since we exist at three levels, it becomes important to understand how to provide the right kind of food or nourishment for all of these levels, i.e., body, mind, and soul.

Objectives

1. How to select the right food or nourishment for the body
2. How to nourish the mind and the soul

Introduction

Food is energy and energy is health.

The necessity of the food for the body

- Food is the external source of energy.

- Our body needs energy (food) for its maintenance, growth, repair, and remodeling processes.

People living without food

There are stories of spiritual people living with little or no food.

There is an authentic story of a lady who stopped eating food forever. It was narrated by Swami Parmahansa Yogananda in the book titled *Autobiography of a Yogi*. It is worth reading.

But an average person cannot live without food for long. One thing should be very clear to all of us: that if we select our food carefully and eat in smaller amounts, we will be much healthier.

Definition

Food is something that nourishes, sustains, or supplies. It can also be defined as the material taken into an organism and used for its growth, repair, and vital processes. It is a source of energy. The word "nourish" means to promote growth or development.

How food becomes our blood

It is interesting to know that whatever we eat, live or dead, organic or inorganic, homogenous or heterogeneous, becomes part of our body tissue. Can you imagine how potatoes, bread, lettuce, eggs, and meat become blood? It is quite a difficult task for the body. All food must be digested and broken down into the very basic ingredients, before it can be converted into blood, and then into body tissue. Let us study the process.

After food is absorbed from the gut it becomes *chyle*. From there on it goes through the certain schema. Ayurveda has given a beautiful description of the schema as follows:

Food is digested > into *chyle* > into *Rasa* (plasma) and lymph > into blood > into muscles > into fat > bone > bone marrow > into semen. Now you should be able to appreciate that semen is the final product of digestion and not just a discharge. (Thus the loss of semen is considered a great loss to one's health, according to Ayurveda and Chinese medicine.)

According to the modern concept, the liver breaks down *chyle* into fat, protein, and carbohydrates at the molecular level, and then these in terms are incorporated into the tissues of the body.

Understanding food

The study of the food is a vast subject. Since food is the cause of health, it is important to understand it thoroughly.

Study of the food groups

There are basically seven groups (classes) of foods: fruits, vegetables, grains, legumes, seeds, nuts, meats, and poultry. Let us study each group in details.

Fruit

Fruit is the essence of everything. Fruit also means results, reward. The fruit of any plant has all of the qualities of that plant, because it is used for the propagation of that species. Vedas states that fruit is the basic food for God. Fruits are served in temples to deities.

The properties of a fruit diet

- It is high in minerals, vitamins, potassium, magnesium, and enzymes. It is also low in sodium and has no cholesterol or fat. Because of the mineral contents, it is good for many conditions of the body, including blood pressure, skin condition, asthma, arthritis, and so on.

- It is the most easily digestible food (extremely important quality), i.e., fruit can be eaten even if one has lost their digestive ability.

- It has a cleansing effect on the system.

- It is a medicine to offset the bad effects of excessive eating, for example, after too many parties or overeating.

- It has a diuretic effect because of the potassium and magnesium in it, and therefore it helps to eliminate waste.

- It is alkaline and anti-mucous (except very few fruits).

- Fruit should not be eaten with carbohydrates, meat, not even with vegetables. Fruit is a meal in itself, and it can be consumed one hour before any meal, for example, breakfast, lunch or dinner, or two to three hours after any meal or in between two meals. Fruit can be consumed with milk. Fruit juices can be acidic, unless they are made fresh and consumed within a matter of minutes. Fresh fruit juice is alkaline. But fruit juice from the market or canned are acidic and can give acidity to many people. A fruit diet also helps arthritis, bronchitis, sinusitis, constipation, and insomnia.

- All berries are rich in iron, phosphorus, and sodium. Lemon juice can be consumed half an hour before each meal as an appetizer. Pineapples, pomegranates, and grapefruit are excellent foods. It is interesting to know that when fruit is in season, it is full of life, is cheapest and also the most nourishing.

- Fruits out of season not only are expensive, but also have less nourishing value. Milk and fruit make a fairly good diet.

- One must remember that fruit has very little protein value. (Whereas vegetables do have better protein value.)

Vegetables

Vegetables can be the root of a plant, stem of a plant or leaves of a plant. For example, roots are potatoes, beets, and carrots. Stems are sugar cane. Leaves are spinach, cabbage, and dandelion.

Fruits and vegetables have different attributes.

They are not the same. While fruits are cleansing, vegetables are building blocks of body tissues. Vegetables not only are rich in vitamins and mineral content, but also have some amounts of proteins. Vegetables can be consumed with any foods including meat. Vegetables can be eaten raw, slightly cooked or steamed. The more you cook, the less is the enzyme, vitamin, and water content. However, cooking makes vegetables easier to digest, so there is a trade-off.

Do not peel vegetables because the highest mineral content is in their outer layer. Aluminum utensils should not be used in cooking because the aluminum is a soft metal and becomes part of the food cooked and ends up in your system.

All vegetables are rich in potassium, magnesium, and calcium. Vegetables and fruits both help in moving the bowels; they act like a mild laxative. They also act as a mild sedative; and therefore help in acquiring a good night's sleep, not only in initiating sleep, but also in maintaining sleep. Fenugreek is good for indigestion. Garlic is good for the blood pressure, heart disease, and arthritis. Almost all vegetables have the quality of being alkaline.

The color of the vegetable is an important factor. The darker the color the better the healing power because of the bioflavonoid content. Yellow vegetables are especially rich in carotene, for example, papaya, yellow pumpkin, and carrots. Red vegetables like tomatoes and cayenne pepper are hot in a nature because the red color represents fire.

Grains

Grains are defined as small hard particles or seeds of a fruit or grass. Grains must be differentiated from legumes. Grains are solid pieces that cannot be split in two, for example, rice, oats, wheat, millet, and barley. These are small and harsh. Grains are excellent sources of protein and carbohydrate, which is essential for our health; however, they lack calcium, and vitamins

The protein content of grains is approximately 10 percent. Grains are rich in sulfur-containing amino acids. When we eat white bread, we lose the mineral content and fiber content. The best way to eat grains is not in the form of white flour but in the form of porridge or whole grain flour, oatmeal, and cornmeal etc. You can also sprout grains (or legumes). The grains are the single most important ingredient of a diet and can amount up to 40 percent, especially if you are a vegetarian.

Legumes or pulses

A legume is any of a large family of plants having fruits that are dry pods and that split when ripe, e.g., peas, pulses or beans. By definition, a legume is that which can be split in two, whereas grains cannot be split into two. Beans are very rich in proteins. The protein content of beans can be as much as 20 to 25 percent. They are also rich in calcium, phosphorus, and iron. While legumes are rich in calcium and lysine, they lack sulfur-containing amino acids. (On the contrary, grains are rich in sulfur-containing amino acids.)

A legume and grain combination is almost a complete food, as both are complementary to each other, for example, wheat bread and beans or rice and beans. Remember legumes and grains are completely absorbed by our system, because these lack fiber, they are constipating by nature. Therefore one should eat grains and legumes with vegetables to avoid constipation. Legumes or pulses are the next most important ingredients after grains and can amount to 5 to 10 percent.

Nuts and seeds

Nuts are also basically seeds. These have high protein content like legumes (10 to 25 percent) and are also very rich in unsaturated fatty acid. These are best for lecithin, vitamin E, phosphorous, sulfur, and calcium. Raw nuts are a rich source of vitamin B complex. These have high caloric value because of the high fat content, but it is a healthy fat, for example, nut butter, peanut butter, or almond butter. This is especially good for people who cannot chew hard foods.

Meat

Since I am a vegetarian, it is very difficult for me to give you sincere advice about meat. But there is plenty of information available on the selection of the meats.

Dairy

Milk and dairy are essential, especially for people who are vegetarian. Milk and meat do not mix in any given meal. Milk preparation includes yogurt, cheese, buttermilk, and ice cream.

Yogurt and buttermilk are very easily digested, and you can eat them even when your digestion is weak. However, because of a cold nature, these should not be taken in excess or when your body is cold. Most cheeses are fermented. Cottage cheese is not fermented. Milk comes in different formulations and preparations including 1%, 2%, free fat, or lactose-free. You should choose the preparation that fits your needs. Ice cream is very rich in fat.

Attributes and the nature of the food

All foods are not the same. Different foods have different qualities, and also can affect the body differently. Here is a list of the qualities/ attributes of foods:

- Rich in protein/fat /carbohydrates
- Vegetarian/non-vegetarian
- Healthy/empty calories (soda, cola, biscuits, candies, alcohol)
- Raw/cooked
- Organic/fertilized
- Natural/processed

- Mucus/anti-mucus
- Acidic/alkaline
- Out of season/in season
- Home grown/imported
- Different tastes of food: salty, sweet, sour, bitter, pungent and spicy (Ayurvedic concept)
- Cooling quality or nature: These foods we love to eat during hot or summer months, e.g., watermelon, cantaloupe, orange, and banana.
- Heating quality or nature: These foods we eat in winter or cold months, e.g., ginger, onion, and garlic.
- Grown underground (potatoes, radishes, ground nuts)/and grown above ground
- Fried food/non-fried food
- Foods that constipate/foods that open the bowel.
- Freshly prepared/stale foods
- Emotional (food prepared for parties or celebrations/food prepared by near and dear ones, for example, mother.
- Spiritual (food served in temples, mosques, churches, and synagogues)

Meta-analysis of all foods

Food is viewed differently by different medical communities

Since food has many attributes, it is viewed differently by various medical communities. Here is a brief summary of some of the concepts. The more you know about the food, the better you can make use of the information for your benefit.

The modern concept

In modern concept, food is classified by calories, protein, fat, and carbohydrates. At times, it may mention something about the fiber content. However, it does not mention the water, mineral, or enzyme content. It does not discuss the freshness, color, and/or the sentimental value of the food. It also does not discuss organic versus inorganic or the acidic versus alkaline nature of the food. It does not mention the taste of the food which the very basic and important concept in Ayurveda.

Nutritionist point of view

Nutritionists view food as raw or cooked, as having water content, mineral content, enzyme content, fiber content, fresh, natural vs. processed, and organically grown vs. grown with fertilizer and chemicals. However they do stress the importance of acidic v*s*. alkaline foods. Still they do not mention the different tastes of foods.

Ayurveda perspective

Ayurveda is big on the prescription of food for each imbalance and/or disease. I have devoted one full chapter on that subject in this book. According to Ayurveda, food is classified by:

- Taste, i.e., salty, sweet, bitter, pungent, and astringent. This is an important and fundamental concept in Ayurveda. Foods of different taste are prescribed based on the different imbalances or diseases at any given time.

- Color: for example, red foods have different qualities than yellow or green foods.

- Fresh foods vs. stale foods have different properties from a health point of view

- Digestibility. How easily food can be digested also impacts our health.

- Nature: Some foods are cooling; others are heating. For example, cantaloupe, watermelon, banana, and some other foods are cooling by nature; therefore they are foods of choice in summer months. Conversely certain foods are heating by nature, for example, peppers, tomatoes, eggplant, ginger, onion, and garlic and therefore are recommended in the winter season.

Other qualities of food

There are other qualities of the food in addition to the ones mentioned above, e.g., vegetarian and non-vegetarian. Certain foods are classified as mucous-producing and some anti-mucous. Therefore you can see that the topic of food is very vast. The idea is to give you some understanding that food has been studied well. We need to create awareness and take advantage of the available information.

Some other considerations

- Food should not be eaten out of season. In other words, in winter you should eat the foods that grow in winter, and in summer you should eat the foods that grow in summer.

- You should not eat many raw vegetables and salads (Ayurvedic concept), especially in winter.

- You should not eat much imported food. Food grown locally meets the needs of the people of that locality.

- Food combinations, i.e., mixing any two animal proteins, are not recommended. This concept is also well known and practiced by the Jewish community.

How to nourish the mind and the soul

So far I have discussed food and nourishment for the body, but it is at least equally important if not more to know, how to nourish the mind and soul. One of the main reasons why people cannot enjoy health and/or happiness is that they do not know or think of nourishing the mind and soul.

A. Nourishment for the mind

The best nourishment for the mind and soul are thoughts that are beneficial, positive, inspiring, and that are based on truth. The source of all these thoughts is our scriptures: Vedas, Bible, and Koran. Being in the company of spiritual people and studying the biographies of great people is also good for the mind and soul.

B. Nourishment for the soul

Spirit is the highest level of life. Spirit must be nourished just like the body and mind. There are special messages/thoughts that are the cause of energy and nourishment for the soul.

Personal level

- Life is continuum and one is immortal.
- One is whole, complete, and free. So one is entitled to bliss in one's life.

Interpersonal level

- We are all interdependent (we need everyone else).
- We are all created equal.
- Love, kindness, and patience make the best spiritual food.

Practical advice and hints

Food and nourishment is the cause of health. In this reference Dr. Henry Beiler states, "Your food shall be your medicine."

You may have heard the sayings, "we are what we eat" and "we eat what we are." So if food is chosen correctly, eaten in the right amount, of the right quality, at the right time, and in the right manner, it can provide good health and longevity.

Right amount

It is important to eat a little less than your capacity. If you feel too full after a meal, it means you have eaten in excess. If you eat food that is not digested in three to four hours, this probably also means that you have eaten in excess of your need. Avoid going for seconds. Going for seconds usually means you are eating too much.

Right quality

You should eat food only for the sake of health and not for taste, fun or for any other reason. Please note that you do acquire the taste of the food that you eat on a regular basis. So once you learn to eat the right quality of food, your craving problem will disappear. Food should be chosen carefully with consideration to its freshness, mineral content, fiber content, and alkaline nature. Balancing the diet is important. You need to eat 80 percent of alkaline food to keep the body alkaline and therefore healthy.

Right time

When you eat is as important as the quality and amount of food you eat. Take the following points into consideration: You should never eat if you are not hungry (very basic principle). Even an average-size meal can be a cause of ill health to a hungry and needy person, whereas the best selected food can be harmful to a person who has a full stomach.

- You should not eat if you are tired. In that case you may drink milk or buttermilk (Prophet Edgar Cayce).
- You should not eat too late at night or two to three hours before going to bed.
- You should not eat too early in the morning, especially if you are not hungry.

Eating a heavy dinner at night and going to bed is one of the contributing factors to obesity, diabetes, blood pressure, GERD, and other problems.

Macrobiotic

Macrobiotic is based on living longer. *Macro* means long; *biotic* means life. Macrobiotic also explains the physical, mental, and spiritual aspects of health. Macrobiotic also explains in what ratio we should choose food.

Following are some guidelines given by macrobiotics:

- Whole grains should constitute 40 to 60 percent of the main diet. Remember grains are rich in sulfur containing an amino acid but are poor in calcium. Examples of whole grains are brown rice, millet, barley, whole wheat, oats, corn, and buckwheat etc. (Grains are extremely important part of our food.)

- Beans and beans products should constitute 5 to 10 percent of the daily food intake. This includes lentils, chickpeas, tofu, peas, legumes, and all kinds of beans. Beans and legumes are interchangeable words. Beans are a very rich source of proteins.

- Vegetables should constitute 20 to 30 percent of your daily food.

- Fruits of the season should be preferred and if possible locally grown.

- All animal products should be eaten occasionally and in minimum qualities.

- Macrobiotics strongly recommends that food should be chewed at least 50 to 100 times for every bite. This not only helps in the digestion of the food, but also one does not overeat. When you do not overeat, you also enjoy the food better. Chewing also makes the food alkaline, because of the alkaline nature of saliva.

Keen observation

Food has a major impact on our health. Some foods affect our system negatively, while other foods affect it positively. At times it can be an individual factor; you should make a note, and use it to your advantage.

The mental and emotional aspect (Ayurvedic concept)

- You should not eat if angry or upset.

- You should observe silence while eating. Do not talk, do business, or make phone calls while eating. (It keeps the mind calm.) It provides concentration and more energy; it also prevents choking.

- You should not take food from an angry or unwilling person, and also you should not cook when you are angry.

Spiritual element

- Give thanks to the provider, the farmer, motherland, nature, and the supreme.

- Eat only your share, not someone else's. It is an importance spiritual philosophy.

- Share food. You should serve others before eating yourself. You should also think of sharing food with starving and hungry people. Sharing food is a great spiritual philosophy and helps the mind and spirit of the person who practices this principle.

The key message

Nourishment of the body, mind, and soul is essential for total health; so it becomes important and pertinent that if you want to enjoy perfect health, you should focus not just on the nourishment of the body, but also the mind and soul.

Mantra

I need food and nourishment for my growth and development. Since I exist at the level of body, mind, and soul, therefore:

- I shall nourish my body with good and healthy foods, after due and careful consideration.

- I shall nourish my mind with positive and beneficial thoughts, so that I can stay calm, relaxed, and balanced.

- I shall nourish my soul (spirit) with love, peace, and happiness.

CHAPTER TWENTY-SIX

Food and Nourishment II (Vegetarianism, the Alkaline Diet)

In this chapter we will learn the pros and cons of vegetarian and non-vegetarian diets. The decision is left to you. I am a vegetarian from birth and so are many people. When people ask me why I don't eat meat, I ask them in return why they eat meat. Vegetarian people often wonder why people eat meat (another life). Non-vegetarian people often wonder how vegetarian people get their protein. Why don't they eat meat? Don't vegetarians miss meat? Some of the questions are strange but some are out of ignorance.

Today people are so focused on protein requirements that they forget the negative aspects of excessive protein or meat intake. They forget that meat is too rich in salt, fat, cholesterol, is acidic and constipating, and also has a mild inflammatory effect.

You must be aware that we do most things in life by habit. Eating is no exception. People who are brought up on rice and fish will keep on eating rice and fish all of their lives. People who are brought up on having three servings of meat per day will continue to do that. Similarly people who are brought up to be vegetarian will continue to eat a vegetarian diet, and so on.

The whole idea of this chapter is to stimulate the thinking process. In other words, you should make healthy choices consciously after careful analysis, and not just by habit.

Objectives

1. A vegetarian diet is complete and healthy.

2. It is the richest source of all minerals, e.g., calcium, potassium, magnesium, and natural vitamins. It is rich in fiber and enzymes. It is also alkaline in nature. Remember an alkaline diet is a healthy diet.

3. Intake of vegetables and fruits is highly recommended and suggested especially for people suffering from high blood pressure, heart disease, cholesterol problem, multiple allergies, skin conditions, osteoporosis, and cancer.

4. Understanding the pros and cons of vegetarian and non-vegetarian diets.

Definition

According to the dictionary, a vegetarian is one that believes in or practices living on a diet of vegetables, fruits, grains, legumes, and nuts. They may consume milk and cheese as animal products but will not eat eggs, fish, meat, seafood or chicken. Eating fish, eggs or chicken is not part of vegetarian diet. Vegans are stricter; they do not consume any animal proteins, not even dairy products.

History

During prehistoric times, primitive man ate mostly meat. He was not knowledgeable in farming or agriculture. Many times he went hungry if he could not find his prey, like most carnivores. But with the advent of civilization, men began to farm and grow grains, fruits, and vegetables. The biggest advantage of farming is that not only is food available on demand, but also one can choose their food at will.

Why a vegetarian diet is the preferred by many

Following are some of the reasons why people choose a vegetarian diet:

Health reasons

A. A vegetarian diet is rich in fiber, alkaline in nature, rich in calcium, potassium, and magnesium, and low in sodium.

B. It normalizes blood pressure. (If it is low, it brings up and if it is high, it brings it down.)

C. It is good for cholesterol and heart disease.

D. It strengthens the bones.

E. It is anti-inflammatory in nature due the bioflavonoid contents of the colored fruits and vegetables.

Religious reasons

Religion teaches us not to harm or injure any life. God is the creator of life.

Emotional aspect

Killing an animal is a violent act. Many people do not want to be a part of that act.

Spiritual reasons

Killing an animal is a selfish act. Spirituality is the opposite of selfishness. It is also believed that the meat of a dead animal has no spiritual energy.

Love of animals

Some people who love animals do not eat meat.

Pros and cons a of vegetarian and non-vegetarian diet

The vegetarian diet

- The vegetarian diet can be complete and balanced with little education and training.

- It is the richest source of all minerals, calcium, potassium, magnesium, enzymes, and fiber.

- The vegetarian diet is the richest source of all natural and live vitamins (vitamin pills are synthetic and chemicals. These are not live and have no life.)

- Vegetables and fruits are alkaline in nature and have anti-inflammatory properties, whereas meat has the acidic quality.

- A vegetarian diet helps not only in inducing sleep, but also in maintaining it.

- A vegetarian diet has a calming effect on the body and mind, and therefore is good for people who are suffering from hyperactivity disorders.

- A vegetarian diet has a mild laxative effect and is therefore good for people who have problems with constipation.

Non-vegetarian diet

- A non-vegetarian diet is incomplete in itself, unless combined with vegetables and fruits.

- A non-vegetarian diet has an excess of salt, fat and cholesterol, therefore it is bad for high blood pressure, cholesterol, and heart disease.

- It (meat) is poor in minerals, e.g., potassium, calcium, magnesium, and others.

- It (meat) is poor in fiber, vitamins, and enzymes.

- It (meat) is acidic in nature and can cause constipation.

- Because of the acidity, meat can cause negative calcium metabolism.
- It also has a mild inflammatory effect.
- Meat also has a stimulating effect on the body and mind and can have negative effect on people with hyperactivity disorders.
- Other interesting observations:

The pig has a very poor memory. When we eat pork, it may have a negative effect on our brain. All carnivores (except scavengers) kill their own prey. Carnivores do not eat the meat of dead animals. Human beings eat the meat of dead animals, but human beings are not scavengers.

Mad Cow disease (a viral infection of the brain of the cow) has been reported recently in literature; it is supposedly due to feeding cows the remains of meat. In Mad Cow disease, there are holes in the brain of the cow. It is believed that is because cows are herbivores, so feeding meat affects their brain in a negative manner. How about humans?

There are many diseases that arise due to eating meat, for example, cysticercosis (from eating uncooked pork, affecting the brain by causing convulsions) and mercury poisoning from fish. Quite often one sees the case of meat poisoning when meat is not preserved properly. It is important to understand that meat rots easily.

Are human beings herbivorous or carnivorous?

The following compares the attributes of herbivorous and carnivores animals. These facts show that human beings are herbivorous by nature:

<u>Jaw</u>

Herbivorous animals have a small and strong jaw, while carnivorous animals have a large jaw for a bigger bite.

Purpose of the jaw

Herbivorous animals need a strong jaw and molars to grind grains and food, while the carnivorous need strong canines and incisors to rip the flesh of their prey. Human beings have a strong jaw and strong molars, not strong canines.

Gut

Herbivorous animals have a large gut for prolonged digestion because vegetables and grains take much longer to digest, whereas carnivorous animals have a small gut because meat rots easily if not digested quickly. (You have heard the same phenomenon if meat is kept out of the fridge, it rots quickly.) Human beings have a large gut that matches that of herbivorous animals.

Tongue

Herbivorous animals have a smooth tongue, while the carnivorous has a rough tongue. Human beings have a smooth tongue.

Perspiration

Herbivorous animals perspire; carnivorous animals do not. Human beings perspire.

Water drinking

Herbivorous animals drink water by lips or by sucking mechanism, while carnivorous animals lick the water with their tongue in order to drink. You know how we humans drink water!

There are others points of difference beside these. When you analyze these qualities, it appears that the human body matches those of herbivorous animals, rather than of carnivorous animals.

Practical points

Most people eat by habit. Please take the opportunity to think today about the advantages and disadvantages of vegetarian and non-vegetarian diets. If you want to become vegetarian, you can do so either gradually or quickly.

If you decide to continue to be non-vegetarian, at least do not eat meat more than three to four servings per week, certainly not more than one serving per day, or at least cut down the portion of the meat to half the amount.

You may give a trial of three to four weeks of being vegetarian and see how it feels. In any event, please eat adequate amounts of vegetables and fruits, as recommended by all health institutes and the American Cancer Institute.

My friend, it is your decision and your choice. Life is an experiment. To become a smarter and better person, you need to experiment with different things. I hope you are open to this experimentation.

Anecdotal case

I have a patient who told me something very interesting. He has a lizard as a pet. He told me that the lizard is a very docile animal if he feeds it only fruits and vegetables. However whenever he feeds it a rat or other meat, the lizard becomes violent for a while. Can meat affect humans in a similar way?

The key message

You should study the multiple positive effects of a well selected vegetarian diet. Certainly you should not eat by habit.

Mantra

I know fruits and vegetables keep the body alkaline. I know that keeping the body alkaline can keep me healthy and prevent many diseases. I also know that meat, cola, soda, desserts, and pickles make my body acidic, therefore I will eat at least five to six servings of fruits and vegetables on a daily basis to maintain my health, but during chronic sickness I will increase the intake of the fruits and vegetables, even further.

CHAPTER TWENTY-SEVEN

Silence: The Opportunity for Mental & Spiritual Growth

In seeking wisdom,
the first stage is silence,
the second listening,
the third remembrance,
the fourth practicing,
the fifth teaching.

—*Kabbalist Solomon Gabrirol*

All man's miseries derive from not
being able to sit quietly in a room alone.

—*Blaire Pascal*
1623-1662

The observance of silence helps you to increase thinking and listening qualities. That in turn leads to mental calmness, clarity, stability, will power, wisdom, spiritual power, and happiness.

All divine knowledge was revealed to rishis (spiritual masters) during the observance of silence and meditation. The power of silence can be sincerely appreciated only by those who observe silence.

Objectives

1. Silence is gift of life. It is the path to wisdom and happiness.
2. Silence at times can be more powerful than words.
3. Learning to practice this art

Introduction

The power of silence

- Silence is a powerful tool for mankind. Silence is essential for learning, thinking, listening, meditating, and concentration, for relaxation, and for increasing mental and spiritual powers. Silence is also essential for increasing the power of imagination and/or visualization.

- Silence is an art of questioning, as well as a technique of answering or replying. While interviewing my patients, when I want to take them deeper into their history, I don't interrupt. I keep looking at their face in silence, which implies please keep on talking, I am listening, and they do.

Let us observe another phenomenon. When we ask a person a question, and they stay silent in response to the question, the interpretation of silence becomes the test of the questioner.

Let us appreciate the effect of the opposite phenomenon, i.e., noise. You must have had opportunities to observe the feeling you get after visiting noisy places, e.g., a rock concert, mad house, noisy factory, home of quarreling people, and so on. All these situations create restlessness in the mind, because everybody gets the color or the flavor of the situations.

Silence can be physical or mental, and these are usually harmonious with each other. Lord Krishna states, "In the life of a yogi, there is an action in inaction, and there is inaction in action."

Definition

As given by *The Oxford Dictionary*: Silence is the complete absence of sound, the fact or state of abstaining from speech, the avoidance of mentioning or discussing something.

Silence vs. meditation

These are two different entities: during silence you use your intelligence for introspection and insight, whereas during meditation you try to bypass your intelligence and focus on stilling the mind to get in touch with the inner self.

A word of caution: Some people, while observing silence, continue to communicate with others either in writing or with sign language. That is not an observance of silence, and it does not have any beneficial effect on the mind or spirit.

Silence observers and appreciators: Silence is everywhere

- My personal experiences as a child, a true story: I was ten years old when my father decided to visit a swami in his ashram, in the city of Jagadhari, (UP) India. He was a well known yogi, and his name was Swami Atma Nand Ji. As we got off the train, we walked to his ashram. As we arrived at the ashram, Swami Ji was sitting under a tree with twenty other saints (spiritual monks) all around him. We bowed our heads and sat down. After one hour we left. No words were exchanged. No greetings. No *namastee*. No hello. No words of any kind. Nobody spoke a word, not us, not Swami Ji, not anyone else. I did not think much of that at the time, but now I think often of that experience and appreciate it.
- There is a group in the United States known as Quakers. Quaker literally means friend. This is how their weekly meeting goes.

They get together in their place of assembly. People come in, sit down, and say nothing. Once in a while, someone may say something of their experience of silence. Generally it is an observance of silence. And at the conclusion everybody leaves. I will call it a spiritual get-together.

- Recently I was listening to Dr. Wayne Dyer. He narrated the incident of his meeting with Swami Ji from India, for which Dr. Dyer had made a long trip. He describes his meeting with Swami Ji as follows. He met Swami Ji for one hour. In that hour both were silent. Both kept looking at each other. Nobody spoke a word. At the end of the interview, Swami Ji asked, "Do you have any questions?" Dr. Dyer said, "No. My questions are all answered."
- Dr. Dyer also narrates the story of Socrates. He had a unique way of teaching his students. Socrates used to tell his students, "Go away from the class and come back after one, two or four hours, whenever you get a new idea." When a student came back, Socrates asked about the new idea, and if new idea was not good enough, he would say, "Go back and think again of a better idea." The message was to try to find the answer within their heart and soul.
- If you look in computer programming, the basic program is 01-01-01-01, and so on. In other words, one alternates with zero. Zero means silence.
- If you analyze music, it has silence alternating with notes in a certain rhythm.

- Swami Dayand of Saylorsburg, Pennsylvania states: "I am silence, you are silence, and we are silence." Please know he is a great spiritual monk.
- Ayurvedic teachers of India are not easy to get answers from. This is not because they refuse to answer, but this is a teaching art. It is like asking the questioner, what do you think? They want to stimulate the thinking by staying silent and looking at the student without answering.
- Dr. James Tyler Kent was one of the greatest homeopathic physicians. He was well known for his teaching art, and it was never easy to get an answer from him. Whenever a student asked a question, Dr. Kent would either stay quiet or say, "Look at such and such chapters or on such and such page." The idea again was to stimulate thinking.
- The Earth is 93 million miles from the sun. There is so much empty (silence) space between the two. It is all silence.
- If you recall the chapter on energy, we learned that there are five elements that go to the creation of the any physical object. Silence or ether (empty space) is the first and fundamental element, responsible for creation of other four elements in this order: ether>air>fire>water> minerals.

Psychology of some people who avoid silence

Many people have not learned about the gift of silence. Others do not want to get in touch with their inner self, because they do not like what is in their hearts. They want to keep away from their inner reality. As soon as they enter their house, they turn on the TV or listen to music or pick up the phone to call someone.

My unique encounter with patients (as a physician)

I often advise my patients that when they come home after a hard day's work, they should rest for five or ten minutes before taking on any chores. In two situations I had ironic responses, which I would like to share with you.

Once I was advising a patient that after she gets home from work, she should not start cooking or eating right away. She should learn to relax for five or ten minutes, unwind from the activities of the day, and then eat or do anything else. When I said that, she started to cry. I asked, "Why you are crying?"

She stated, "If I stay quiet, I become miserable, because I can't think of anything except my nasty job and my nasty boss." Now I could understand her pain and emotional state as to why she wanted to keep herself occupied.

I gave the same advice to another patient; when she comes home from work, she should rest for five or ten minutes before she does any chores. She told me that she is so afraid of entering the house, as if something is hiding in her closet or in a dark corner of the house, in spite of searching everywhere. In other words she is fearful at all times. She must turn up the volume on the TV so loud so that she would not think of anything else. She does not want to think about life. She wants to live the life of TV or radio. She even keeps the TV on all night during sleep. In her own statement "I watch TV while I'm awake, but the TV watches me while I'm asleep" It is really a sad story.

The inner self should be the source of solace, joy, and peace, and not of misery.

Multiple benefits of observing silence:

1. It increases the thinking and listening quality.
2. It increases mental calmness.

3. It increases mental clarity.
4. It fosters mental stability.
5. It increases will power.
6. It helps you grow spiritually.
7. You become wiser when you observe silence.

Practical points

In the beginning you can begin to observe silence for four hours a day/per week. After you become accustomed to four hours, then you can increase to twelve hours, and then to twenty-four hours a day/per week. Or you could observe silence two hours a day on a daily basis or make a habit of observing silence on weekends, or any of the above combinations. At least do one thing, do not talk unless it is called for, or it is absolutely essential.

One question

Can you think of anything that is so easy, so effective that does not need any investment of time, money or anything else, yet increases mental clarity, mental balance, and spiritual growth? I hope you come up with the same answer as I did: nothing. My friend, think it over. It is one of the cheapest and best gifts.

The key message

Silence is one of the easiest and cheapest ways to increase thinking and listening ability. It also increases mental clarity and wisdom. It does not require investment of time or money. It also does not require any training, and it does save time.

Mantra

I understand by observing silence, I can increase my intelligence and wisdom. I will observe the practice of silence on a regular basis. Today I can start the practice with as little as one hour a day with a fixed time schedule. For example, I will not speak from 9 o'clock to 10, or 3 o'clock to 4, or any other time, whatever does not interfere with my work schedule. At least I shall talk in my daily life when it is absolutely necessary to talk.

Silence is Everywhere and in Everything

Everything comes from silence
Everything goes to silence
Everything is silent
Silence is everywhere and in everything

Silence marks the beginning
And the end of everything
Silence is everywhere and in everything

I am silent
Silence is in me
He is silent
Silence is in Him
Silence is everywhere and in everything

CHAPTER TWENTY-EIGHT

Meditation: Connecting to the Bliss Center

Why meditation?

You all know the power of your mighty mind. It wanders, travels, imagines, and does all sorts of things. It can drive you crazy and wild. In other words it can control your life. Do you agree?

Now if you want to control your mind instead of being controlled by it, you meditate. With meditation the mind calms down. It gets its rest. You become more relaxed and more alert. This is the power of meditation.

We all blame our mind for being restless or for going into thousands of directions. I believe it is unfair to blame the mind for this. It is just keeping up with the busy universe.

Tell me one thing in the universe that is stationary. Everything is on the go, on the move, on the run. Certain things move at such a speed that you cannot comprehend. It makes you feel dizzy. How often do people say slow down, stop, let me rest, let me pull myself together?

Look at how our Earth revolves on its own axis approximately one thousand miles per hour. It also revolves around the sun 1.8 million miles per day. Other planets — Mercury, Venus, Mars, Jupiter, Saturn, Uranus, Pluto, and Neptune — have similar patterns, some going faster than others. Coming back to Earth, even air, water, and fire are in motion. If you study the little atom, you will be amazed to know how its tiny electron is in continuous motion for its survival.

People often get impressed with a juggler in the circus throwing certain objects into the air at a certain speed and rhythm. It is not a big deal. You and I can do it with a little practice. The magic would be if someone could make a ball stop in the air! Look at the power of a good speaker or writer who makes you freeze with his words or a magician who makes you spellbound with his tricks.

To make things stationary needs power. Similarly to make the mind stop needs power, real power. Now appreciate the power of a meditator (yogi) who can make the body stationary for days or months. They can stop eating for months. They can stop breathing for months, because they know how to make the mind stop and rest. To me it is real magic, and everybody loves magic.

Now you can appreciate another power of meditation. The spiritual masters who have meditated for years and years have developed special spiritual powers. One saint appeared at two places at the same time. It is a true story. Another saint was buried alive for six weeks underground and when disinterred (unearthed), he woke up as if he had been sleeping. Another saint saw the dead body of a child who had just died. He asked the people not to cremate the child. He suddenly collapsed and died and the child woke up. This is an authentic story narrated by Swami Yoganand Pramahansa. This all demonstrates the attainment of the power of our eternal spirit through meditation.

Objectives

1. To understand the science, philosophy, and benefits of meditation
2. To learn the art of meditation

Definition & Introduction

According to *The Oxford Dictionary*, meditate means to focus one's mind for a period of time for spiritual purposes or as a method of relaxation.

Literally meditation means to think or measure. However, meditation is anything but thinking. As a matter of fact, during meditation one is advised *not* to think, so as to bypass their intelligence or conscious level. The reason is that to get into the deepest state of meditation, one has to enter the subconscious mind. The subconscious mind does not think or reasons, so it is important to block the thinking or conscious mind during the period of meditation.

Swami Paramahansa Yogananda has defined mediation in his book titled *Man's Eternal Quest* as follows:

> "Meditation is becoming one with the soul. It means banishing the consciousness of being related to the body and to the human limitations, and trying to remember that one is a soul. When man begins by the conscious mental effort to relate himself with the immortal soul, rather than to the body that he inhabits for one life only, he will recall more of his past life experiences and will eventually remember that he has come down from the bosom of God. In him lies the memory of all the experiences of one's life and of all lives. When man communes with the soul within the forgotten times and the power of deathless, self will come back into his consciousness. In summary, meditation means to remember that one is not a mortal body, but an immortal soul, one with God."

It is very interesting that Swami Vivekananda has explained the same philosophy in a different version. Swami Ji states:

> "Meditation has been laid stress upon by all religions. The meditative state of mind is declared by the yogis to be the highest state in which the mind exists. The mind of an average man when studying the external object identifies with it and loses him/herself. This is the problem."

To use the simile of the old Indian philosopher:

> "The soul of man is like a piece of crystal, but it assumes the color of whatever is near to it. Whatever soul touches...it takes its color. That is the difficulty. That constitutes the bondage. The color is so strong, the crystal forgets itself and identifies itself with the color. Suppose a red flower is near the crystal and the crystal takes the red color and forgets itself, thinks it is red. We have taken the color of the body and have forgotten what we are."

He further stresses that "we are lost in this world because we have forgotten that we are souls."

He further writes:

> "All our fears, all worries, anxieties, troubles, mistakes, weakness, evils are from that one great blunder—that we are bodies. This is the ordinary person. It is like a person taking the color of the flower near to it, we are no more bodies that the crystal is the red flower. As the practice of meditation is pursued, the crystal knows what it is, takes its own color. It is meditation, which brings us near to the truth than anything else."

Stages of meditation

Swami Ji describes the three stages of meditation: Dharna, Dhyana, and Samadhi. The first stage is called Dharna, where one tries to concentrate the mind upon an object, say, a glass of water, excluding every other object from the mind except this glass, but the mind wavers.

In Dhyana, the second stage of meditation, the mind becomes strong and does not waver so much. Then there is still a higher state when the differentiation between the glass and oneself is lost; this is called Samadhi or absorption. Now the mind and glass are identical. One does not see any difference, all the senses stop, and all of the power that has been working through all the channels of other senses is focused on the mind. This glass is under the power of the mind entirely. This is to be realized by the meditator. This is meditation.

Meditation vs. silence

One needs to differentiate between the two; these are two different entities. In silence one uses one's intelligence for introspection and betterment of the self. In meditation one has to bypass their intelligence or the conscious level, so that they can still the mind and appreciate the real nature of the self; that is, one is eternal, complete, and free. (See Chapter 21)

Meditation vs. prayer

Meditation and prayers are both good and useful. However one should be clear that meditation is several times more powerful and more effective in balancing the mind and strengthening the soul than prayer.

How meditation works

It is accepted and known fact that the real source of bliss resides within the heart and soul of each and every one, but because of our busy life we forget ourselves and get entangled up in the world. The more and more we get entangled, the more and more we get lost and forget that we are eternal blissful souls.

It is like the story of the boy who goes to college to get a degree. But in college, he gets into bad habits and gets distracted from his real mission. As a result, he does not graduate and he fails. Now he feels frustrated. This is a story of an average man in the school of life.

Let us take another example. You must have observed that on a cloudy day, you can neither appreciate the rays of the sun in the day time, nor the beauty of the moon and stars at night. Similarly on a foggy day we cannot even see ten feet away. Here clouds are metaphorically used to express the confusion or lack of clarity of the mind of a busy life.

If you observe a swimming pool where people are swimming, the bottom of the pool is not clearly visible. But the moment they get out of the pool, you can appreciate the clarity of the water and see the bottom of the pool. If someone loses something in the pool while people are still swimming, it will not be easy to find until people stop swimming. So is the state of your busy mind.

Similarly unless and until you still your mind, you cannot appreciate your real nature, i.e., you are the soul, not the body. Here the motion of the water is metaphorically used again for a busy life.

Control your thoughts: enjoy the bliss

Controlling your thoughts is the first and most essential step in the process of meditation and to get the desired result. The thoughts of a busy life can take the mind in a thousand directions. The importance of controlling of your thoughts is also essential for rest, relaxation, and balance of the mind. Let us see how it works. For the sake of understanding let us compare our thoughts with ocean waves.

You may have experienced that on a quiet evening the gentle rhythmical waves of the ocean are soothing to the body and mind. However, if waves pick up speed and intensity because of the wind and the fullness of the moon, they can become noisy and make you nervous. If there is a hurricane, ocean waves can become violent and threatening. You may want to run home.

Our thought process affects our mind and body in a similar manner. A person with a calm mind has their thought process under control. These thoughts arise in a rhythmical and controlled fashion.

However, thoughts of an aggressive and negative quality can make a person nervous and agitated or even restless. Such is the effect of thoughts on the mind.

Remember your mind creates one thought per every one to one-and-a-half seconds. That means about 60,000 to 80,000 thoughts per day. By each practice of meditation, the thought process begins to slow down. As that happens, the mind becomes calm and relaxed, while staying more alert. This unique combination of staying alert while being relaxed has multiple advantages. It increases concentration and clarity and expands consciousness.

Please remember: The mind of a meditator is relaxed, calm, at peace, and yet is very alert.

Benefits of meditation for the body, mind, and soul

The advantages of meditation are directly related to the degree of attainment of the stillness of the mind, which is directly and proportionately to the time spent in meditation.

Physical benefits

1. The pulse rate goes down.

2. The heart rate slows down. The heart spends more time in relaxation vs. in contraction, thereby prolonging the life of the heart.

3. Breathing becomes deep and slow, and therefore one needs to take fewer breaths and thus life gets prolonged. (See Chapter 10)

4. The face becomes lustrous, the aura improves, and one attracts others.

Mental benefits

1. In the very beginning, you start to feel calm and at peace.
2. Concentration increases.
3. Intelligence increases.
4. The mind becomes more balanced.

Spiritual benefits

1. The consciousness expands.
2. In the last stages of meditation (Samadhi), one attains a state of blissfulness.

Preparation for meditation

1. Sit calmly for a minute or so.

2. Think that one is healthy physically, mentally, and spiritually.

3. That one is fortunate because one knows this esoteric knowledge and can use it for one's benefit.

4. That one is blessed, being able to relax and have peace.

5. That one is not the body, but the immortal soul. Think on this phrase constantly.

Point of Focus

Some techniques use an external object as a point of focus, i.e., a candle, mirror or any object. In my opinion, this is probably not the ideal way, because one needs to focus deep inside, not outside the body. The most advanced techniques use the point of focus within the body, e.g., mid-forehead (the middle of the eyebrow), crown chakra (top of the head) or medulla oblongata (back of the head).

Technique (as explained by Swami Vivekanand)

1. Get in any position/posture where you can sit for a long period of time.

2. It is preferable for you to meditate at the same time and same location, if possible.

3. Sit straight and close your eyes.

4. Start breathing deeply and slowly. Now continue to breathe deeper and deeper. (The technique of slower and deeper breathing stimulates the parasympathetic nervous system, making one relax.)

5. Focus the mind on the mid-forehead or crown chakra or medulla oblongata. Choose one spot only.

6. Stay in this state for at least three to five minutes and keep breathing deeply and slowly.

7. Start chanting the sound of the word Aum (OM) focusing on the letter M rather than letter A or U.

8. Do it for several minutes.

9. Go to a whisper sound for several minutes.

10. Now start mental chanting; no whispering, i.e., no audible sound should be produced.

11. If you stay in this stage, you will go into subconscious chanting where you find peace, and finally you will merge with the supreme which is the source of all happiness and bliss.

Authentic story

Here is a true story of Anand Swam Ji, a great yogi who had reached the peak stage of meditation (Samadhi). He states:

> "Once I was meditating for three-and-a-half hours, and I was so much absorbed in my meditation that I was lost completely in myself. My guru Ji wanted to test me, and he put a nail in my leg to test the depth of Samadhi, and he states that I did not feel any pain or discomfort of any kind, because I was totally with my soul, not with my body."

It is possible to reclaim that state during meditation. Many yogis have achieved that state, and I have had the fortunate experience of meeting with such saints. What a joy to meet these people!

Joke

When a hen sits on eggs for days without moving in order to provide comfort and heat to the eggs so that they can hatch, what does she do? Does she meditate?

Caution

Meditation is a path to spirituality; its results are rewarding in the least. The benefits are at every level of the body, mind, and soul. Learning meditation without its practice is of no use. It is only the practice that provides the benefits. Practice must be done on regular basis. If you can try it for a month or two, then it would be easy to convince yourself of the positive effects of meditation. (Please give it a fair trial. It is my humble request. You will thank yourself.)

If you are a meditator already, you should thank a million times to the person from whom you have learned this special gift of life.

Patience is a virtue

We need patience everywhere and anywhere in our life. But probably there is no other field where patience is more needed than in the practice of meditation. I often hear people complaining after a few weeks of meditation that their mind is still wandering and they cannot focus. However true it may sound, it is not true.

The beneficial effect of meditation starts from Day One. The mind begins to slow down from Day One. The reason people do not perceive in the very beginning is because the mind is in the habit of going in a thousand directions. With each practice of meditation, one or two directions get less, but are not appreciated by the beginner. So don't give up. Rest assured you will get there. You are not wasting your time. The results of meditation are cumulative.

The key message

We are the soul and not the body. The soul is the seat of all joy, peace, and bliss. Meditation is a technique that helps us in the realization of this goal.

Mantra

I understand that all joy and bliss of life resides within my heart and soul, and not outside. I will meditate regularly to make my mind more calmed, more relaxed, and more alert, so that I can enjoy the state of blissfulness.

CHAPTER TWENTY-NINE

Yoga: The Harmonious Working of the Body, Mind, & Soul (Spirit)

Nothing exceeds the excellence of man
who is the combination of the body, mind,
intellect, and the atma (soul).

Na hi manushat shreshthataram hi kinchit maha bharat.
Vedas

What is yoga and how can it bring joy into one's life? To appreciate that, one needs to know that one of the golden truths of life is that:

All the peace, joy, happiness, and bliss of life resides within everyone's heart and soul, and not outside.

For this realization, or to reach this state, you need the harmonious working of your body, mind, and soul. When these elements are in harmony with each other, you become whole. Everything is in unison. This is what I mean by harmony. This is what I mean by yoga.

Harmony equates to cooperation, coordination, and smooth functioning, which leads to growth, success, and happiness.

Wherever there is harmony, there is union, peace, success, and joy. Conversely wherever there is disharmony, there is pain, misery, and failure. It is true everywhere and anywhere, whether it is at the level of the body, mind, families, organizations, government, country, world, or even the whole cosmos.

Simply said
Balance of the mind> harmony of the body mind and soul > union of the body mind and soul > wholeness > bliss of life. This is yoga.

Upanishad explains yoga as follows: Yoga means union with the self or the supreme. Union with self means that the physical, mental, and spiritual components of the individual are in harmony with each other. This happens only when one is balanced and healthy at all three levels; then one is in touch with the inner self. It is then only that one becomes content, peaceful, and attains bliss.

Bhagavad Gita glorifies yoga as follows: "The tongue cannot describe the happiness that communion with the self (or God) brings, when the ignorance and other like impurities have been washed away by the means of yogic Samadhi, and the self rising within itself concentrates on God."

When you meet a person whose face is lustrous, who is happy and joyous, who is calm, content, and at peace within the self, and emanates peace to others, you can consider that person a yogi.

In this reference let me ask you an intriguing question. The vast majority of the people – and you may be one of them – search joy and happiness in the outer world and fail again and again. Yet nobody dares to look differently or into a new direction. Do you know why? You may continue to think of the answer to this question, as you continue to learn about yoga in this chapter. Let us continue……..

Objectives

1. Understanding yoga, the philosophy and technique
2. Yoga is for each and every human being. It is not just for the monks or spiritual masters.

Introduction

The word "yoga" is derived from Sanskrit word *yuj* meaning to join or come together. The English word "yoke" has the Sanskrit root. A yoke is a wooden stick which joins two oxen together while working in the field. Literally speaking, yoga is used when two things join together. Generally yoga means union of the soul with God. But for people who do not believe in God, getting in touch with their inner self can also be called yoga. When all three levels of our being – physical, mental, and spiritual – are in harmony with each other, we become complete and whole. This is yoga.

Definition

According to *The Oxford Dictionary*, yoga is a Hindu spiritual and ascetic discipline, a part of which includes breath control, simple meditation, and adoption of specific bodily postures.

Patanjalli states: "Yoga is the complete and ultimate control of all mental activities," or *yoga-schitta-vrtti-nirodhah.*

Lord Krishna in *Gita* states: "Yoga is maintenance of emotional equilibrium in adversities, as well as in favorable circumstances (*samatvam yoga Uchyate*)."

Behold the statement of Swami Vivekananda, how he describes in depth the characteristics of yogi: "The one who finds in the middle of intense activity the greatest rest, and in the middle of greatest rest intense action is a yogi. Yogi can attain that highest state of mind which is super concentration."

Philosophy of yoga: How does it work?

Every species produces its own kind. The orange tree produces only oranges. The mango tree produces only mangoes. Since we are the children of divine God, we must be divine by nature. The divine does not suffer. The divine does not die.

You ask why human beings suffer. According to *Upanishad*, when human beings lose their self-identity or self, they suffer. To simplify it further, when human beings bond or become attached to the temporary and mundane issues of the world, they also become temporary and mundane. Thus they lose their eternal nature and suffer.

The state of the mind of such suffering human beings can be compared with the state of the mind of the "lost child." Here I will narrate the classical story as it depicts the state of the mind of the lost child. The story goes as follows:

A child goes with his mother to a fair. The child asks his mother for a balloon, but his mother refuses to buy one. As they walk few steps further, the child asks for a candy but the mother again refuses to buy any. The mother keeps on walking. Then the child asks his mother if he can go on a ride, but somehow his mother also refuses. All of a sudden the child gets detached from his mother and gets lost and starts crying. His mother also gets restless looking and searching for him. People take pity and try to comfort and console the child, but he does not stop crying. People offer him balloon, candy, rides, but he refuses everything and does not want anything. He continues to cry and states, "I want only my mother." Suddenly his mother finds him. Now he starts laughing. He clings to his mother. Now he gets a balloon, and he is very happy with it.

That is our state of affairs. Our mind is restless and wandering, because we are lost and isolated from ourselves and from the Lord, and hence we suffer.

Yoga is an art and science that helps us to connect with the inner self and the mother (or the Lord). This is where all the peace, contentment, joy, and happiness lie.

Preparation for yoga

It is common knowledge and understanding that to have union with somebody the following criteria must be met:

1. Both parties must be willing and desirous to meet.

2. The date, time, and place to meet must be set.

3. For a true union one must have a common agenda. In other words, one has to come to the same frequency and same wavelength as the other being, i.e., both must have a common ground.

So far okay. Let us go deeper.

God is willing and desirous to meet us. Are we? If that is the case, one problem is solved. Next, we must set the date, place, and time. Again that is not a problem, because He is available to us now and always, as He loves us so much. He is ready any time, any minute, and any place, but we have to be ready. Are we ready?

Next is the agenda. This is the most critical element. As I have expressed earlier, to have a true union we must have a common agenda, i.e., we must feel, think, and act like the other being. We must try to understand Him and His teachings and come to the same frequency, same wavelength, and same tune that He has. This is a very real secret for the true and happy union. He is energy, love, kindness, forgiveness, truth, sincerity, and justice. Are we like Him? We have to think carefully before we go to see Him. We need to try to match His tune and His energy level. At least we should try our best, and then He will know that we are trying hard to meet Him.

Let me give you a few examples to show you how important it is to come with the same frequency and same wavelength with the person to whom you are going to meet.

When we go meet a business man, we dress nicely. We have our checkbook, important papers, a nice place to meet, and we are ready for business. When we go to meet a friend for a tennis game or a golf game, we have to dress like him; we need to have our tennis racket or golf club and balls, sporty attire, and we meet him in the club or golf course. When we go to meet an athlete, we dress like an athlete, we want to have extra water to drink and several hours to spend, and then we are ready for the game. When we go to meet a swimmer, we must have swim clothes, meet at the swimming pool, and be ready to go.

When we decide to go to temple or church or go to meet a spiritual master, we take a shower and dress in simple and clean clothes (no fancy or sporty clothes). Now good and positive thoughts come to our mind, and we are ready to go to the temple/church or to meet the spiritual master.

Similarly to meet God, we have come to the same frequency or same wavelength or tune that He has.

History of yoga

Yoga is a contribution of the seers or spiritual masters of India. The spiritual master who made it a philosophy and a science with clear direction is known by the name of Patanjalli Rishi, who lived 200 B.C. All branches of yoga follow Patanjalli yoga.

Yoga: some misconceptions

Yoga has been misunderstood by some people, including many teachers of yoga. The misunderstanding has been that yoga means *asna* or postures or, at the most, postures plus meditation. It is not true, although *asna* and meditation are part and parcel of yoga, but are not yoga in totality.

Yoga is a science and art which has eight developmental stages. All of the eight stages are essential for perfect physical, mental, and spiritual transformation.

Four branches of yoga

The aim of yoga is self-realization which is equal to God's realization. There are four branches of yoga and all have same common goal. One can choose any one of these or any combination of.

<u>Dhyana or Raja Yoga (yoga of meditation)</u>

This is essentially meditation. It is a science and art of meditation. The mind is restless, fleeting, and wandering in nature. When we meditate, our mind becomes focused on one point, and we begin to appreciate the real joy, peace, and contentment within ourselves.

<u>Karma Yoga (yoga of action)</u>

When a man helps others without seeking any reward for self, he is said to be karma yogi. He becomes like the Lord and starts to perceive Him within the self. This is exactly what God does. It is popular with people who love to help their fellow beings.

<u>Janana Yoga (Yoga of knowledge)</u>

In this branch of yoga, a man seeks truth by means of intelligence and logic. This is in favor with people who are philosophers or who tend to think in a logical manner.

Bhakti Yoga (yoga of devotion)

Here the devotee surrenders himself totally at the feet of the Lord. He loves God as his mother. Mother is the most reverend word in the dictionary. This branch is a favorite with people who are very simpleminded, emotional, and devoted to God. Here one gets rid of their ego and totally merges with God.

Science of yoga: Eight stages

The science of yoga, as laid by the Patanjalli Rishi, consists of eight stages. Therefore it is known as Astanga Yoga (*asta* means eight, *anga* means steps). These are as follows:

1. Yama, (moral conduct), five in number
2. Niyma, (physical and religious observance), five in number
3. Asana, correct postures to still bodily restlessness
4. Prana Yama, control of *prana*, subtle life currents and mind
5. Pratyahara, interiorization
6. Dharna, concentration
7. Dhyana, meditation
8. Samadhi, the ecstasy of oneness with God/or with self

Yama (5) and Niyma (5) are 10 commandments to build up moral and ethical observance and physical discipline. Unfortunately and sadly many yoga teachers who are not well versed with yoga philosophy ignore these commandments completely. These commandments are so important that even if one does not practice other stages of yoga, these virtues alone can grant happiness, peace, and stability of the mind; hence it is a prerequisite for self-realization or yoga.

Stage 1: Yama or restrains (the moral conduct, principle of self-control) – Five Commandments

Non-violence

This is the principle of co-existence with all. To love every human being and not to think, say, or do badly. The biggest advantage of this principle is that the sense of enmity (malice) towards all creatures disappears from the mind. Jealousy is considered a violent act, according to Vedas.

Truth

To speak the truth to whatever is seen, listened to, read, and inferred in the mind. The advantage of speaking the truth is that when people speak the truth, they become respectable and trustworthy with every being that they meet.

Abstention from theft

Not to take anything from anybody without permission, in thought, speech, or action. By such a practice a person achieves spiritual qualities. Vedas says if the thought of stealing comes to one's mind, even if one does not steal, one is a thief in a real sense, although one may not be a thief in the public's view.

Celibacy

To protect physical powers, one should not waste semen. One must read one's scriptures. The advantage of celibacy is that one's mind, speech, body, and intellect become strong.

Renunciation

No hoarding, no storing harmful and unessential objects, or thoughts. The advantage is that one rises to a spiritual level, and one realizes who they are.

Stage 2: Niyma or self disciplining: five commandments

Purification of body and the mind

Purification of the body is easy: keeping it clean, taking a bath, and eating healthy food. Purification of the mind means to tell the truth, study religious books, practice religious conduct, and so on. The advantage of this stage is that the mind remains concentrated and cheerful.

Satisfaction

To be satisfied with whatever is gained in the form of pleasure, teaching, power, wealth, and so on. The advantage being that one is happy, content, and at peace with the self.

Penance (Tap)

Not to get upset with hunger, cold, heat, loss, gain, and other dualities of life. The advantage being that one becomes strong and in charge of their own mind.

Self-study, reading of the Vedas or other scriptures

Study and knowledge are essential for mental and spiritual growth and development.

Ishwar-Pranidhan (surrender to God)

To accept God's gift and surrender to God completely

Stage 3: Asana (yoga postures)

The mind and body are deeply and directly connected with each other. Not only does the mind have an effect on the body, but the body also has an effect on the mind. You may have noticed that children who suffer from hyperactivity mental disorder not only have a restless mind, but also has a fidgety body. By the practice of Asana, the body and mind start working in coordination with each other. The body and mind calm down; such is the value of Asana.

Stage 4: Pranayama

Pranayama is disciplining Prana, the subtle energy which pervades and controls all of the functions of the body. Pranayama is a special method of breath control with which the life force is brought under control. This is achieved by controlling the incoming or outgoing breaths. The results can be further intensified by reciting the word OM while doing the

Pranayama. Further Pranayama helps to bring involuntary actions such as respiration and heartbeat under voluntary control. It takes practice to achieve the desired results. How does one control prana? It is a technique of deep and slow breathing, while keeping the mind focused on the breath. To understand more clearly let us study the act of breathing.

The act of breathing: four components as follows:
The first component consists of the act of inhaling (breathing in), which should be very deep and very slow. The second component consists of holding the breath in as long as one can comfortably do so without any discomfort. The third component consists of exhaling the breath very slowly. The fourth component consists of holding the breath out as long as possible without any discomfort.

In a nutshell, each act of inhaling and exhaling should be a slow and deep process. Each act of breathing out should take twice the time than that of breathing in. For example, if you take ten seconds to inhale, then you should take twenty seconds to exhale. Or if you take five seconds to inhale, then you should take ten seconds to exhale. Further you need to focus that each act of breathing in is energizing to the body and the mind, and each act of breathing out is relaxing to the body.

There are different names given to the different acts of breathing in or breathing out, but that is not important. These names are as follows:

- *Purak*: This is the way of drawing in breath slowly and deeply to your full capacity.

- *Stambhak*: This is retention of the breath (either holding it in or out).

- *Rechak*: This is the way of letting your breath out slowly and to the maximum capacity.

Importance and advantages of Pranayama

1. The mind becomes stable.

2. You become more intelligent.

3. The pulse and heart rate slow down, so the heart has more time to relax and will have a longer life.

4. You need fewer breaths per minute. Number 3 and 4 cause prolongation of life.

5. Some yogi have mastered and controlled their breaths to the extent that they can hold their breath up to twenty-four hours or more, and can suspend their life force during that period.

Stage 5: Pratyahara (sense control)
In Pratyahara one withdraws the attention from external sensory stimulus by redirecting the attention inwards. In the beginning, you develop discipline over your appetite by controlling your hunger, and you discipline the feelings of lust through divine support. Also Pratyahara includes the appropriate nutritious intake of vegetarian food to achieve longevity and a healthy life by disciplining the mind over sensual desires. It is a stage of introspection, redirection, and arousal of inward energy. Pratyahara paves the way for improved focus and voluntary restraint of the emotions, the higher wakeful state of inner self, and the consciousness; this leads to satisfaction and contentment.

Stages 6, 7, and 8
These three stages are one step after another from the basic level of Dharana to the highest level of Samadhi.

Stage 6: Dharana
Meditative concentration

Stage 7: Dhyana
Intense meditation, complete submersion in meditation

Stage 8: Samadhi
Transcendental absorption of consciousness with the absolute, infinite, divine super-consciousness, and to experience the bliss of the union

Test of mental and spiritual growth and development

This test is based upon the first two stages of yoga: Yamas and Niyamas.

This test not only helps you to facilitate the understanding of the first two stages of yoga, but also gives you an opportunity to test yourself on a regular basis as you travel on the path of yoga. This test was originally devised by a great swami. Thanks to him. He would not like to be credited, so his identity is not disclosed. Are you ready for the test?

The Yamas – Restraints

AHIMSA – NONINJURY: I harm others by thoughts, words, or deeds.

1. Never 2. Rarely 3. Sometimes 4. Often

SATYA – TRUTHFULNESS: I refrain from lying and betraying promises.

1. Always 2. Usually 3. Sometimes 4. Rarely

ASTEYA – NONSTEALING: I steal, covet or enter into debt.

1. Never 2. Rarely 3. Sometimes 4. Often

BRAHMACHARIYA – SEXUAL PURITY: I control lust by remaining celibate when single or faithful in marriage.

1. Always 2. Usually 3. Sometimes 4. Rarely

KSHAMA – PATIENCE: I restrain intolerance with people and impatience with circumstances.

1. Always 2. Usually 3. Sometimes 4. Rarely

DHRITI – STEADFASTNESS: I overcome non-perseverance, fear, indecision and changeableness.

1. Always 2. Usually 3. Sometimes 4. Rarely

DAYA – COMPASSION: I conquer callous, cruel and insensitive feelings toward all beings.

1. Always 2. Usually 3. Sometimes 4. Rarely

ARJAVA – HONESTY: I renounce deception and wrongdoing. 1. Always 2. Usually 3. Sometimes 4. Rarely

MITAHARA – MODERATE APPETITE: I eat too much or consume meat, fish, fowl or eggs.

1. Never 2. Rarely 3. Sometimes 4. Often

SAUCHA – PURITY: I avoid impurity in body, mind and speech.

1. Always 2. Usually 3. Sometimes 4. Rarely

Your total score for the Yamas: _______

The Niyamas – Practices

SANTOSHA – CONTENTMENT: I seek joy and serenity in life.

1. Always 2. Usually 3. Sometimes 4. Rarely

TAPA – AUSTERITY: I perform sadhana, penance, tapas and sacrifice.

1. Regularly 2. Often 3. Sometimes 4. Rarely

DANA – CHARITY: I give charity without thought of reward.

1. Always 2. Usually 3. Sometimes 4. Rarely

ASTIKYA – FAITH: I believe firmly in GOD, Gods, guru and the path to enlightenment.

1. Always 2. Usually 3. Sometimes 4. Rarely

ISVARAPUJANA – WORSHIP: I cultivate devotion through daily worship and meditation.

1. Without fail 2. Often 3. Sometimes 4. Rarely

MATI – COGNITION: I develop spiritual will and intellect with a guru's guidance.

1. Always 2. Often 3. Sometimes 4. Rarely

SIDDHANTASRAVANA – SCRIPTURAL STUDY: I study the teachings and listen to the wise of my lineage.

1. Very often 2. Often 3. Sometimes 4. Rarely

HRI – REMORSE: I am modest and show shame for misdeeds.

1. Always 2. Usually 3. Sometimes 4. Rarely

VRATA – SACRED VOWS: I fulfill religious vows, rules, and observances faithfully.

1. Always 2. Usually 3. Sometimes 4. Rarely

JAPA – RECITATION: I chant holy mantras daily.

1. Always 2. Usually 3. Sometimes 4. Rarely

Your total score for the Niyamas: ______

Total score for both Yamas and the Niyamas: _________

The lower your score, the farther advanced you are on the spiritual path and less help you need to get on the right track. Take this test as often as you need to gauge your progress.

Here are your categories based on your combined scores:

20: Saintly person	50: Average struggler
25: Spiritually adept	55: Karma's slave
30: Advanced meditator	60: Bad example
35: Devout pathfinder	65: Selfish brute
40: Serious seeker	70: No one's friend
45: Good soul	75: Devious scoundrel

80: Dharma's (Religion's) enemy

Yoga's contribution towards physical, mental, and spiritual health and happiness

1. Your mind becomes clear and pure: This is the result of the first and second steps of Yama and Niyama.

2. Yoga improves coordination of the body and mind: the reward of Asna, the third stage of yoga.

3. Yoga helps to balance your mind: the first three stages of yoga plus paranayam.

4. Yoga helps you feel contented and satisfied: the reward of the fifth step of yoga known as pratyahara.

5. Yoga helps to improve concentration and the intense concentration: the reward of the sixth and seventh stages of yoga.

6. Through yoga, you achieve union of the body, mind, and soul, the reward of the last stage of yoga known as Samandi, i.e., union with self or the supreme. Now the consciousness expands, and you realize the real eternal nature of the self. You begin to enjoy the bliss of life.

Additional benefits

1. Your face becomes lustrous.
2. Your body becomes symmetrical.
3. You can control your heart rate and breathing.
4. Your intellect becomes sharp.
5. Your concentration becomes intense.
6. You begin to have true and beneficial thoughts.
7. Your consciousness expands; you feel content and blissful.

The key message

The regular practice of yoga creates harmonious relationship between your body, mind, and soul. When that happens, you realize that you are whole and complete. Thus you do not need anything anymore. You have it all. This produces the deepest level of contentment and bliss: yoga.

Mantra

I will stay focused on the harmonious working of the body, mind, and soul to create a perfect balance in my life.

CHAPTER THIRTY

Art of Eternal Happiness: Always Calm, Always Smiling

I want happiness. You want happiness. Everyone wants happiness. This is the first and foremost desire of everybody. No one would argue about that. If you take that a step further, it is also the blessing of our parents, elders, gurus; even the Constitution of the country is written for the freedom and happiness of all.

I have also come to a realization in the mature years of my life. A person who is not happy in life should not consider him/her self a successful person, irrespective of what else he/she may have attained in the form of education, college degrees, wealth, family status, and social status etc.

You should also know that happiness cannot be linked to wealth, education, social status, or anything else. You know some poor people are happy; others sad. Some educated people are happy; others sad. Some wealthy people are happy; others sad. In other words, you see happy and sad people in all walks of life.

The reason why I equate success to happiness is because people who cannot fulfill the first and foremost desire of life, i.e., to be happy, what else will they achieve in life? You will also come to another realization after reading this chapter; that happiness is with us and was always with us, but we have gone crazy looking for it somewhere else. Let me remark here that:

I love, respect, and honor happy people, because to me these are successful people, and everybody loves success.

A warning to miserable and unhappy people: Please understand one fact clearly, that you can blame only yourself and no one else for your own miseries and unhappiness. Conversely, if you are living happily and are upbeat, you can credit yourself.

The importance of happiness can be understood by the following little incident. This is the story of a swami (the spiritual monk) of the highest caliber. His name was Swami Dayanand Sarswati, a guru. He was the greatest humanitarian of his time. One day he was asked by the people why he works so hard for the well being of the society that he has no time to take care of himself. He replied: "The mission of my life is that I want freedom and happiness for the whole humanity and not just for myself."

I have also observed and it probably will stand the test of the time: A wise person is a happy person, and a happy person is a wise person. The wise person faces the difficulties and challenges of life in a calm and balanced manner. They do not lose themselves and continue to sail their lifeboat. Conversely the ignorant person becomes the victim of the difficulties and challenges of the life. They may lose themselves or even sink their lifeboat.

I also like to quote His Holiness Dalai Lama in this reference:

> "Today you have all the ingredients of happiness. You don't need a better career, a better wife, more money, better job, or better opportunities. You have everything right now, at this minute to be internally happy."

In other words, happiness can be ours today without any change in the external world. Happiness lies within the heart and soul of every being; the only thing required of you is to peek within.

Please devote yourself fully to the study of this chapter. It may change your life. Are you ready?

Objectives

1. Happiness is the desire, need, and want of every being.

2. Furthermore if one is not enjoying the life of freedom and happiness, one can only blame oneself and no one else.

3. It is important to understand that happiness is a learnable art and science. I shall show you how.

4. For happiness, one does not need anything more than what one already has. The only thing required is to change the way one looks at things and at one's life.

Introduction

Some people know the art of living. They enjoy life. They are happy people. They make themselves at ease in most or all situations and circumstances. They are pleasant to deal with. They have a balanced state of mind. They are calm and content. They are a joy to be with.

It is not that they don't have problems in life, because life comes with problems, but they have decided not to be victims of their problems. They know how to deal with problems effectively as these arise. Or you can say that they keep their problems in proper perspective.

One more thing that happy people believe in is brotherhood and sisterhood, and they have a broader view of life, compared to the selfish and narrow view of unhappy people.

Definition

The Oxford Dictionary defines happiness as a feeling of strong pleasure and contentment; or willingness to do and accept anything, or being fortunate and lucky. One may want to know that there are certain terms, such as happy as the sand boy, slap happy, or happy as a clam or happy go lucky. These terms denote only short-term happiness. This is very different from lasting happiness that we are talking about in this chapter.

Laughing is not happiness. Laughing is definitely good for health. Even foolish and miserable people can laugh at times, but they may not be happy. Animals can neither laugh nor be happy.

Eternal happiness can be best defined as the ability to maintain a state of happiness under all conditions and circumstances, which is the result of the balanced mind and strong spirit.

Behold what Vedas states in reference to happiness: happiness is the prerequisite for salvation.

How Vedas defines salvation: Each and every person without exception has to face difficulties and challenges of life, because these are part of normal life. Those who are strong mentally and spiritually can face the problems and difficulties in a calm and balanced manner and become victorious. They do not become victims of the problems of life; hence they find freedom, happiness, and finally salvation.

Happiness can be studied in degree, intensity, and duration. Duration is more important than intensity, because our life is for eternity.

Please note that health and happiness are related and allied words. They vary in degree and/or intensity. Health means sound physical and mental health, whereas happiness means sound physical and mental health, plus contentment and adeptness. The last two words, contentment and adeptness, are added to the definition of health and are indications of spiritual health.

One should also be clear that long-term or eternal happiness can be provided only by the things/conditions or situations that are long-lived. Therefore money, position, power, social status or anything that is short-lived cannot provide long-term happiness, whereas our soul (with its companion mind) is for eternity. Hence anything that strengthens and benefits the spirit can provide long-term happiness.

Why seek happiness?

It is a general principle of life that we search for only those things which we owned at one time or other. We do not search for those things that we did not own before. In other words, we must have been the owner of happiness at one time or the other. Remember how happy and carefree we were as little children? As we grew older we lost that quality. This is the reason we are searching for the same joy and happiness. As a matter of fact, happiness is our real innate nature that is with us from birth.

Learning from the different behavior and characteristics of happy and unhappy people

Let us learn from the characteristics and behavior of happy people.

<u>Personal level</u>

They have a balanced state of mind.
They are calm by nature.
They have deep contentment in life.
They are at peace with the self.
They have good analytical ability with foresight.
They have an appreciation of life.
They have an ability to enjoy life as it is (without any precondition).
They accept life and its events as temporary and natural.
They have higher or highest goals or missions.
They have a good listening ability.

They appreciate the fact that two opposite conditions and situations generally coexist, e.g., day and night, health and disease, pain and pleasure, success and failure, honor and insult, birth and death, etc.

<u>Interpersonal level</u>
They work on getting rid of the ego.
They are pleasant to deal with.
They have a comforting and helpful nature.
They have love and compassion for others.

Now analyze the characteristics and behavior of unhappy people.

<u>Personal level</u>
They have an unbalanced state of mind.
They have wandering minds.
They are restless and impatient.
They are poor listeners and have short fuses.
They are shortsighted.
They complain about life, people, and situations.
They have low goal and ambitions.

They are discontented and dissatisfied with things, people, situations, and possessions.
They are unable to enjoy life, as if they are waiting for something good to happen.
They feel like they are a victim of every misfortune in life, e.g., pain suffering, illness, etc.
They are ignorant about life, e.g., they do not understand life, have poor analytic ability, and poor knowledge about the self.

<u>Interpersonal level</u>
They have imbalanced egos, either feeling very special or at the bottom.
They are unpleasant in their dealings with others.
They are selfish in nature (a telltale sign).
They are only for themselves and do not care for others.

Having said that, let us compare and contrast the characteristics and behavior of happy and unhappy people for ready reference:

Happy People = HP Unhappy People= UNP

Upbringing
HP – Usually good upbringing
UNP – Poor upbringing

Art and Science
HP – Constantly searching for happiness
UNP – No such vision

Seat of happiness
HP – Know that happiness lies in the heart and soul, not outside
UNP – Look for happiness in the wrong places and the wrong things, i.e., money, position, power, spouse, and family

Focus
HP – Focus on positive events, people and aspects of life
UNP –Focus on negative events, people, and aspects of life

Mind
HP – Healthy and balanced state of mind
UNP – Flickering and unstable state of mind

Energy
HP – Positive energy and positive aura
UNP – Negative energy and negative aura

Behavior
HP – Pleasant to talk to, predictable behavior
UNP – Moody (unpredictable behavior)

Appreciation
HP – Appreciate everything they have
UNP – Complain about everything they do not have

Contentment
HP – Content and satisfied with what they have
UNP – Neither content nor satisfied, no matter what they may have, because they want more and more

Complaining
HP – Usually doesn't complain about anything, accept people and situations as they are

UNP – Complain often about their job, the weather, their spouse, their friends and families

Equal Rights
HP – Believe in equal rights
UNP – Do not have this concept

Opinion
HP – Respect their opinions, as well as those of others
UNP – Dogmatic and force their views on others/or may even downgrade others' viewpoint

Success and failure
HP – No success and failure; it's life. If they fail, try again.
UNP – Failure is final outcome. If they fail, it is all over.

Interdependence
HP – Believe and understand we need each other and are interdependent
UNP –Believe people need them, or the opposite, they feel that they are dependent upon others

Altruism
HP – Respect and care for others
UNP – Selfish and indifferent to others

Acceptance
HP – Do not like to argue and are open-minded
UNP – Argue and likely to get into fights, don't accept others or others' viewpoints, make enemies easily

Life Outlook
HP – See life as challenging, make the best of it. It has roses and thorns.
UNP – Life is pain, suffering, and thorns.

Anxiety and Worry
HP – Don't worry about anything unnecessarily.
UNP – Spend so much time in anxiety and worry that hardly any time is left for anything else

Fault-Finding
HP – Focused on improving their weaknesses, strive for continuous improvement for a happier life

UNP – Focused on weaknesses of theirs as well as of others, with no clue or efforts on improving

Take Responsibility
HP – Take responsibility for whatever happens, good and bad
UNP – Blame others for any misfortune or negative outcome

Truth
HP – Tell the truth
UNP – Lie and keep secrets

Ego
HP – Give up their ego, everyone is equal without exception. We are just numbers.
UNP – Have problems with their ego, think they are very special and indispensable, or believe they are not worthy of anything

Expectation
HP – Don't expect anything from anybody, expect from the self
UNP – Expect too much from others, often a cause of anger and frustration

Dependency
HP – Do not depend upon others
UNP –Depend so much upon others, that it can become a cause of failure

Life's View
HP – Have better understanding of life
UNP – Have no concept of life

Result and methods
HP – Focus on the right path and not so much on the results/outcomes
UNP – More focused on results and rewards, not on right or wrong.

Focus
HP – Focus on solving the problems
UHP – Focus on counting the problems and the difficulties

Happiness and unhappiness - analysis

- Causes of unhappiness and the solution
- Test – Are you a happy person?
- On the scale of happiness – Where would you fit?

- True story

Causes of unhappiness and the solution
Unhappiness is based on the diseases and/or weaknesses at the physical, mental, and spiritual levels.

Most people are aware of only the physical diseases or weaknesses. The average person has no concept or does not understand mental and spiritual diseases and weaknesses that can cause diseases; although it is the latter that is the main cause of misery and unhappiness.

Physical level	Mental level	Spiritual level
Diabetes Arthritis Asthma High Blood Pressure Headaches Neck Pain Back Pain Constipation Indigestion Difficulty Breathing	Sleeplessness Depression Sadness Mania Forgetfulness Indecisiveness	Selfishness No concept of life No understanding of life Meanness Argumentative Quarreling Anger Fears Greed Jealousy Hatred

Solutions
Inasmuch as weakness and imbalance are the cause of all diseases and suffering, conversely good health and strength at the mental and spiritual levels is the cause of all freedom and happiness.

The Test: Are you a happy person?

I devised the following test based on my knowledge and experience. It gives good insight about oneself.

I am usually calm in difficult and challenging situations. Y/N

I am fairly content within myself. Y/N

I usually make good decisions and choices. Y/N

I usually do not have to repent for the decisions and choices that I make. If I make a wrong decision, I accept it and then try to fix it. Y/N

I take responsibility for all of my actions/outcomes. Y/N

I do not blame others for any negative outcomes and their results Y/N

I am open-minded. Y/N

I respect my opinions and also those of all others. Y/N

I avoid arguments and quarrels. Y/N

If you have answered most of the question with yes, then you are a happy person. Congratulations! Otherwise it is the time to inquire deeply for an understanding of life. You may also read the chapter again.

The Scale of happiness - Where do you fit?

Happiness and unhappiness are at opposite ends of the spectrum; hence there is a big gap between the two. The majority of people fall into this gap; probably you are one of them. Now appreciate the two extremes:

Always happy (perfect mental balance)
Mentally balance (good or okay)
Slap happy
Normal
Sad
Depressed
Unhappy, miserable

Now try to analyze to which category you are close. Pause! Take your time. You can try to analyze others as well in this reference. This is only to improve your own understanding. You know that no one has any right to judge anyone else.

True story

This is about one of my patients, V. S. She is 48 years of age. She is a pleasant person and nice to work with. She has a mature and stable mind. I asked her about her family. She replied, "I come from a family where everybody is angry or miserable. Nobody is happy. Everyone complains. However I learned something from it. I said to myself, this is not the life that I want. Now I am a happy person. I am content. I feel God is with me. I believe everything is happening the way it is supposed to be."

This magical transformation came to her life because she made her decision. Magic can happen, but you have to make the decision first. Are you ready for such a decision?

Practical points and lessons

After having said so much, let's review some practical tips. I have classified all these hints into six sections:

1. General
2. Personal level
3. Interpersonal level
4. Difficult situations and suffering
5. Personal experiences/favorites
6. Law of nothingness

<u>General</u>

1. Happiness is here and now. Nobody knows about tomorrow. Tomorrow could be the same, better or even worse. Most likely it would not be much different from today, unless one does something about it. Why wait for tomorrow? Today one has everything that one needs to be happy. One is the owner of a powerful mind and an eternal and holy soul; that is all one needs to be happy.

2. Having good thoughts is probably one of the single most important secrets of a happy life. Good thoughts are the basis of good words and statements. Good words lead to good actions. Good actions make one strong mentally and spiritually, and a strong mind and spirit is the basis of happiness. (Conversely bad words or actions have exactly the opposite effect).

3. Every action produces a reaction which is equal and opposite. Be aware what you say or do. Everything will bounce back to you. Every positive word and act will bring a positive effect, and every negative word or act will bring a negative effect. This is the law of nature.

4. The right path is more important than the outcome or the result. A happy/wise person will follow the right path even when the outcome may not be so favorable. On the contrary an ignorant person may focus more on the results. They may use even unfair or foul methods for which they may have to suffer. (*Bhagavad Gita)*

5. It is very important to take the responsibility for one's actions and/or results (good as well as bad), because it provides one the opportunity to fix the problem. Blaming others is counter-productive and even dangerous. When one blame others:

   a. One loses their friends and even can make enemies.

   b. One says indirectly that they are not going to do anything about it. Why should I? I am not responsible for it, therefore no change or improvement. Same old story continues.

6. Contentment is another important secret. There is no end to needs, desires, and wants. You can do this experiment. First, try to increase all your desires, wants, and needs for certain duration, e.g., one to three months. Now try to decrease your desires, wants, and needs. You will learn something from it. Please give due consideration to this thought. Contentment does not mean you should not make progress on a daily basis, but that you should not break down if the reward is not appropriate or proportional for the work.

7. Today is the time to appreciate. We are given this beautifully engineered body with a good brain, good vision, hearing, smell, and taste. Each one of these elements is worth a lot of money. We are also given sharp intellect, a good mind, and an eternal soul. These are priceless. We are all surrounded by loving parents, teachers, friends, and well wishers. Don't forget that the Earth, moon, stars, and galaxies are for our benefit as much as are the air, water, fire, and minerals, and so on. If we take the time to appreciate them, then the outlook on life can change for many.

8. Every truth strengthens the mind and the spirit. Every lie weakens the mind and the spirit. Whereas weakness is the cause of pain and misery and strength is a cause of joy and happiness.

9. Life can be full of surprises; don't be shocked by them.

10. Everything is even in the end. There are no losses or gains in life. You leave the world empty-handed, the way you came. So calm down and relax and enjoy life (*Bhagavad Gita*)

11. Remember things could be much worse than they are today. (Please give this statement serious thought.)

12. Relatively: Everything is in a relative phenomenon. Nothing in the world is 100 percent good or 100 percent bad. If you keep analyzing and thinking deep enough what happens is this: what you thought once was so good now it does not sound that good; equally what you thought once was so bad, now it does not sound so bad. Think about it.

13. Time: Live in the present. Look ahead and move forward. Forget the past. Nobody has seen the future. Time is the best gift of life. Do not waste it. Time is running out. (*Bhagavad Gita*)

<u>Personal level</u>

1. Ego: Get rid of it. We are just a number in this world. You have to trust me on that. I am saying this emphatically. One may be the most important person in their judgment or even in the company of their friends, coworkers, or family members, but in the opinion of all others (which is close to 6 billion people) each of us is just a number.

2. Neither control others nor be controlled by others. (Teachings of scripture)

3. Helping others is a reward in itself. Remember it is only healthy and strong people who can offer help. And people who attempt to help others also become strong. One should also not hesitate to ask for help when in need. It is one of the principles of happiness (*Bhagavad Gita*).

4. Understand our enemies: We need to realize that our worst enemies are not our spouse, boss, children, friends, or anything external, but

our own internal enemies, such as anger, greed, jealousy, hate, fear, and worries. These accompany us day in and day out, 24 hours a day 7 days a week. They eat, sleep, and walk with us. They are the causes of our unhappiness and weaknesses. We need to control them for our happiness. (*Bhagavad Gita*)

Interpersonal level (dealing with others)
Dealing with others people is one of the biggest challenges of daily life and is a test of one's mental and spiritual strength.

Few hints:

1. Do not attempt to change people. If you will try, you will fail; take it for granted! Change happens only when one is willing and determined and not before that. You can't change anyone nor can anyone change you.

2. Difficult people are like poles and walls. Please do not strike them, unless you want to break your head.

3. Avoid argument convincing and confrontation.

4. Express your views clearly and candidly and leave the rest to the individual.

Diseases, difficult situations, and suffering

1. One must be very clear that these are as much a part of each and everyone's life as are health, joy, and happiness.

2. Nobody, including you and me, is exempt from these.

3. These also provide an opportunity to deal with the challenges of life and to become victorious.

4. Every victory takes one to a higher level or at a higher path. All the great peoples are such examples.

Just think how all of the greatest people on Earth without exception have suffered and suffered immensely; whether it is Lord Buddha, Jesus Christ, Mahatma Gandhi, Lord Krishna, Lord Rama, Swami Dayanand or anyone. It appears from the above as if suffering is essential to rise up in life.

Personal experiences/favorites

The following are some of the points that have helped me the most. They are for your consideration and thoughtfulness. They may or may not be applicable to you.

- Acceptance

Probably this is one of the best lessons in life. Everybody is okay. You and I are okay. Everything in life is okay. Everything that will happen or is happening is also okay. Every situation and every life event is okay and is part of life. Nothing is that good or that bad. Accept and relax. (*Bhagavad Gita*)

- Ego

When I finally realized that I am nobody special, I began to feel at ease in the most difficult and odd situations.

- Exposure:

Avoid or at least cut down the exposure time to people who are miserable and unhappy; they could be your coworker, spouse, colleagues, and so on.

"Law of Nothingness"

I do not believe there is such a law. However, today I am making such an announcement. This law is extremely beneficial and has important implications in a person's life. The benefits of the law can be understood by the fact that anyone who will attempt to analyze, understand, and inculcate the message of this law into life will find ease at heart and peace and joy in the life.

You will appreciate that the word "nothing" is also used quite often in day-to-day language. For example, when you ask people what they are doing, and if they are not doing anything important, they often say, "Nothing." Similarly, you must have observed that when you ask people what is this or that, and if it is not important, they often say, "It's nothing." Here nothing means not important or insignificant. Nothing does not mean zero.

Now please try to understand the depth, the meaning, and the message of the twelve components of the law and see how much of this you can apply in your life for your benefits. Next are the twelve phrases or the components of the law of nothingness. These are:

- You come from ***nothing.***
- You go to ***nothing.***
- You came with ***nothing.***
- You go with ***nothing.***
- Assume ***nothing.***
- Presume ***nothing.***
- Judge ***nothing.***
- Expect ***nothing.***
- There's ***nothing*** that good in life.
- There's ***nothing*** that bad in life.
- If you keep thinking on any idea deeply and long enough, you can create something from ***nothing.***
- An ignorant person can make a mountain of ***nothing***, and an intelligent person can convert the mountain into ***nothing.***

Thank you for taking time to study the law of nothingness.

The key message

My dear friends: Please listen and listen carefully. This is your life and a long one. You can make it simple, pleasant, and enjoyable, or you can make it tough and miserable. It is all your choice. It is all within your power. Remember if you will make it simple and enjoyable, it will be good for your heart and soul, and it will make life easier. Think about it. Take a pause!

Also understand that if you cannot be happy today, I do not see how you can be happy tomorrow or the day after or in a month or year after (or even in the next life, if you believe in reincarnation), because things are not going to change unless you do something about it.

Now, would you like to read this chapter again with open eyes and an open heart?

Mantra

If you recite, read, sing this mantra three times a day for one month the first thing in the morning, it should become part of your life and hence change your life for the better.

I am strong and in charge of my life. This is the way it's going to be.

With the power of my mind I can make any issue, any situation, any time, or any person as big or as small as I wish.

I feel confident that from now on I will be able to handle any situation, circumstances, or person in a calm, relaxed manner.

From now on I shall enjoy the life of relaxation, freedom, and happiness.

Life is very long, so it is better for me to enjoy it.

Life is a game that one must learn to play

Life is a game that one must learn to play
If one plays it right, it shall be a happy game
Or it can be all misery and pain
Life is a game that one must learn to play
If one plays it right, it will be a happy game

If there is an unhappy ending
One must think with the mighty brain
Where am I wrong and what is wrong?
Don't ever think, who else is wrong
It is my life and I am the boss

Do not ever blame the spouse, or the friend
Or it can be all misery and pain
Life is a game that one must learn to play
If one plays it right, it will be a happy game

Happiness is now and here
Don't need to go anywhere
Happiness resides within the heart and soul
Search and find yourself
Don't go crazy like deer musk
Or it can be all misery and pain
Life is a game that one must learn to play
If one plays it right, it will be a happy game

Tomorrow things may not be any different,
But one must learn to play it different
You better learn this game of life
Or it can be all misery and pain
Life is a game that one must learn to play
If one plays it right, it will be a happy game

Happiness is the desire, need, and want
Our parents, teacher, scriptures, and constitution
Have similar want
Try to understand the need, and not the want
Or it can be all misery and pain
Life is a game that one must learn to play
If one plays it right, it will be a happy game

Happiness is a sure sign of success
One must be clear about this concept
Don't try to find happiness in money, position, or fame
Or it can be all misery and pain
Life is a game that one must learn to play
If one plays it right, it will be a happy game

Happiness is a learnable art
It is no special craft
Nobody is born that smart
Better understand this life's game
Or it can be all is misery and pain

Life is a game that one must learn to play
If one plays it right, it will be a happy game

Think what you need today and tomorrow
Not what you could need tomorrow
Look what you have
Not what you could have
There is no end to need, desire or want
Keep the contentment, the only want
Or it can be all misery and pain
Life is a game that one must learn to play
If one plays it right, it will be a happy game

Pain and suffering are part of life
It belongs to every human life
Day and night cannot be separated
Summer and winter are brother and sister
Good and evil often co-exist
Health and sickness are not exempt
Understand that you are part of this game
Or it can be all misery and pain
Life is a game that one must learn to play
If one plays it right, it will be a happy game

Pain and suffering are special events
It is an opportunity to get better or best
So that you can pass the final test,
If you fail this test of life
It can be all misery and pain
Life is a game that one must learn to play
If one plays it right, it will be a happy game

This life looks very short,
But we know the soul has no death
And life is an eternal process
Staying on the right path is the final test
So that one can get home (heaven) safe and sound
This is really not so complex
Try to understand the game of life
Or it can be all misery and pain
Life is a game that one must learn to play
If one plays it right, it will be a happy game

Make friends; make friends, oh my bhai
One never knows when one needs these brothers or bhai
In this, or even the next life
Because life is a continuous process
Without a sister, brother, or a friend
It can be all misery and pain
Life is a game that one must learn to play
If one plays it right, it will be a happy game

Anger, hate, jealousy, greed are animal creatures
They kill and eat every brother and sister
These creatures make enemies day and night
One ends up with no brother and sister
When one reaches its final home (Heaven)
There will be no one to meet or greet
So better get rid of these creatures
Or life can be all misery and pain
Life is a game that one must learn to play
If one plays it right, it will be a happy game

Happiness is not in money, position, or fame
These are just temporary names
When the body is healthy and intelligent sharp
No one can make one fall apart
When ego is balanced and intellect keen
When the mind is calm and the spirit strong
When the heart is love and the voice is sweet
One wins the game of life
Time is now to understand this game of life
Or it can be all misery and pain
Life is a game that one must learn to play
If one plays it right, it will be a happy game

Make the heart pure and the mind strong
Good words and good acts are the best plan
This is the summary of the final plan
Call me Brother, Singhal, Doctor or Pratap
But take my heartfelt advice
If one want happiness and freedom of life
You better understand the game of life
Or it can be all misery and pain

Life is a game that one must learn to play
If one plays it right, it will be a happy game

CHAPTER THIRTY-ONE

Young Forever: Always Good, Always Young

Nobody wants to die, and nobody wants to get old. Is this not true? Yes! Of course it is true! There is some truth behind it. Let us see what it is.

We have already discussed that we are souls and souls do not die, hence we are eternal. If we are eternal then there is no question of dying. Now about getting old, the question of age is only in one's head and mind. Read Chapter 1 on how to slow down/reverse the aging and disease process; most of your questions about aging will be answered.

Let us go a little further into this subject. Everybody wants to feel and look young, and why not? It is all within our scope. We love young people with young minds and young spirits. Being young also makes us feel good. Being young also signifies health, vigor, beauty, freshness, and joy.

Objective

To understand that it is within the power of the mind of each and every individual to stay young, irrespective of chronological age

Definitions

To make the reading a little interesting, let us define certain terms:

Age: According to *The Oxford Dictionary*, age is defined as "the length of the time that a person has existed."

Child: A young human below the age of full physical development

Young: Having lived or existed for a short time

Youth: The period between childhood and adulthood. It is defined with the quality of vigor, freshness, and immaturity. (Notice the word immaturity is attached to the word youth.)

Old age: The later part of normal living, associated with experience. (Notice the words experience and maturity are related and linked to the aging process.)

Understanding age: a new perspective

We must remember this very basic concept that we exist at three levels, i.e., body, mind, and soul. The body represents only a part of us, and thus is not us. If you want to count age in reference to the body, then you must know that there is not a single tissue in the body that is more than two years old, no matter how old you may be. If you want to count your age in reference to the mind, then it is purely the mind's game. We are as young or as old as our mind thinks. If you wish to count the age in reference to the soul, then you must know that the soul has no age. It is eternal just like nature and/or God. Therefore we are eternal and always young.

You also need to know that age and time are relative terms. We count time or age from certain events, e.g., birth, graduation, marriage, death, or anniversary. Now if you wish to take the subject of biological or chronological age, you should know that chronological age is also a relative term. People count their age from the time of birth. Is that a true definition? Think about it. Some people at forty behave like they were sixty; while others, at forty, act and behave like twenty. So you can see that even at the age of forty, there can be a difference of twenty years. Is it not amazing?

Age: Positive and negative outlook/reaction

People act and react differently to different situations and events. Age is no exception to this rule. The difference can be vast. Some people take everything in a positive manner, while others take everything in a negative manner. On birthdays some people get overjoyed, celebrate, do parties, and get a kick out of it. While for others, it is a day for sadness, negative stigma, and a day to hide. They may even cry if someone congratulates them on their birthday. Is it not a game of the mind?

You should also know that some people lie about their age. Do you know why? There is some philosophy behind it. So let us take a look. Some people at forty will say that they are thirty or even younger. I believe these people have an inner weakness or low self-esteem that they want to hide. While others at age of sixty will say that they are seventy and eighty years old. These people want to impress you as to how good they look and how well they have maintained themselves.

Should I tell my age to others?

This has been a topic of discussion with many. However, one great swami has advised that one should not tell their age. But I personally believe that you should do whatever you are comfortable with. There is no magic or math involved in this.

Authentic story of a swami

Once I was interviewing a great swami, who was sixty-five years old. I asked him how old he was. He replied joking, "I am only thirty-five." I knew Swami Ji does not lie. I asked him how that is possible. He replied, "I became a swami at the age of thirty, so the first thirty years of my life were wasted, and I don't wish to count those years."

Benefits

Remember our existence is at least at three levels: body, mind, and soul. There are several other levels of existence but these are not important at this juncture. Now appreciate the age of your body, mind, or soul.

Soul

If you believe you are the soul, then you are eternal and forever. Therefore there is no need to count age. You are always young. Does it not make you feel good?

Mind

If you believe you are the mind, then it is a mind game. You are as old or as young as you think. Then why not always think and act young.

Body

The topic of the body is very interesting. If you read thoroughly Chapter 1, you must understand that our body tissues are constantly renewed, rejuvenated, and restored everyday. The reason people look old is because they believe they are getting old. The interesting and practical fact is that the aging process can be reversed by healthy habits and mental attitude etc. (See Chapter 1).

To stay in good shape and health, you must:

A. Exercise the body, mind, and soul. (See Chapter 24) Exercise can make you ten to fifteen years younger physically, mentally, and spiritually.

B. Nourish the body, mind, and soul for a longer life. (See Chapters 25 & 26)

C. Rest and relax at the level of body, mind, and soul. (See Chapter 23)

D. Stay on the right path. This contributes greatly to making you feel young and happy.

E. Meditate: Anyone who meditates regularly can easily look and feel fifteen to twenty years younger.

F. Mind: Life is the game of the mind, and age is no exception. Therefore think, talk, dress, walk like a young person and you would feel young.

G. Probably the best thing to do is stop counting your age, because you are an eternal soul and always young. And that is the truth!

Test

What is your age? You can choose one or more answer.

A. I am ______ years **OLD.**

B. I am _______ years **YOUNG.**

C. I am as old as I think.

D. I am eternal, and hence forever.

Key phrases

Think, talk, act, dress, walk like a young person. Always say I feel good and young! Eventually this will start to sink in.

Mantra

I will keep myself young by training the mind to think, act, and feel young. I am the eternal spirit (soul). I am young in my feelings, words, and acts.

Young

I am young
Because my mind is young…

I dress like young
I eat like young
I sleep like young
I walk like young
I dance like young
I am young
Because my mind is young…

I talk like young
I laugh like young
I think like young
I am young
Because my mind is young…

My body is young
My soul is young
I am young
Because my mind is young…

Young are you
Young is he
Young is she
Young is this whole world
I am young
Because my mind is young…

CHAPTER THIRTY-TWO

Transformation: The Magic, from Here to There

If I told you that you can create magic in life, would you believe it? Yes, it is true and you had better believe it. The word magic has several definitions. But the important definition applicable here is to make it very good and enjoyable or of enchanting quality.

We see so many magical things every day that we do not appreciate because they are either slow or very slow motion, and hence fall into the range of expectations. We call it magic when things happen suddenly, e.g., when a magician makes balls disappear or when a lady in the box changes into a tiger.

Now look at the magic of life. Every day we see babies or new life appearing on this planet. And also people disappearing (dying) for good. Not only this, but at times they reappear at another places or at other times (reincarnation). How about the cancer patient getting rid of the disease permanently or thieves or robbers becoming monks, swamis or priests? Is it not magic?

When a failing student goes to the top the class, is it not magic? Behold your body. Your mighty heart cannot rest for even one moment from the time you are born. Is it not magic? The power of the human brain is bigger than any computer in the world. I could give you thousands of such examples. But the real amazing thing is that we do not get amazed by all these happenings, yet we do get amazed by the magician making balls disappear (just an illusion). Does it make any sense?

When we read, hear or watch stories of great achievers in any field, whether in the field of math, computers, science, literature, poetry, astrology, medicine, engineering or even in the spiritual field, such as prophets, rishis, and so on, we get amazed. Our mouth remains open! Our eyes don't blink! Our body feels the surge of energy! And we want to do something. The new hope enlivens us. Is it possible? Can I do it? Yes, anybody can do it. These were ordinary people like you and me, except that these people had the desire, determination, and will to do something. They were the followers of their own chosen path. These people faced the difficulties and challenges and evolved in life.

This teaches us only one thing: that every human being is born with great potential and with the magical powers. And it is never too late to use that potential/power.

Objectives

1. One must realize their potential. The sky is the limit. One must have determination for whatever they wish to achieve.

2. However, if one cannot be a great achiever, at least one should be able to live the life of health, happiness, and freedom. I believe this is not expecting too much from an average human being.

Introduction

Human beings are the most intelligent creatures on Earth. They have more information, knowledge, tools, equipment, and software than ever in the history of mankind. This is how and why we rule the Earth and even some planets.

Transformation – Step by Step

Transformation is an active process. It is not a passive phenomenon. An average person lives passively. They do not see, hear, think, or analyze in reality. They say things because others are saying it. They do things because others are doing them, whether they are right or wrong. They see misery and suffering yet they do not try to understand how and why. They do not even try to understand themselves. Such is the degree of ignorance!

They are living for the sake of living. They spend all their life making a living (money) until they cannot make a living any more, either because of disease or death. To some people this is life. Would you call this life? This is a very passive life. Real life is energy. Energy is action.

Let me give you some insight by examples:

<u>Animal life</u>

The life of a dog, cat, rat, bird, fish, cattle, or any other animal is fixed in a predictable manner. Everything is like automation, like machines. They are living machines. They are born, have offspring, and then die.

<u>Life of very average humans</u>

They have a pretty predictable life pattern, not much different. They are born, go to school, may or may not go to college, get a job, get married, have children, and make money until they cannot make anymore, as if the only purpose of the life was to make money, either for themselves or for their children. They face the miseries of life with sadness and depression or even some good times here and there. No betterment, no real progress mentally or spiritually. No real joy or happiness. And then it is time to say goodbye to this life! Could we call them living machines? Is that living? Is it really so different from the animal life?

Life of slightly higher level human beings

People in this class may be better than the first category, but not so much better. I am sure you can do better than them. These people have made some transformations. They have focused on education, college degrees, post-graduation, and professions. Still a lot of tension, hard work, struggling, family feuds, and that's how they die. No real joy or maybe joy here and there.

One must be clear that school education, college degrees, and diplomas are only for the sake of making a living. These do not provide happiness. Happiness is based on mental balance and spiritual growth that one does not learn in school or college.

Life at a still higher level

These people are happy and content. They have found peace in their heart and soul. They feel the joy of life. They are healthy at the mental and spiritual levels. Their mind is balanced. They remain balanced and calm in the face of difficulties. They have learned from every difficulty and challenge of life. This is a very basic achievement of a person as prescribed by our scriptures. So they die in peace.

Life at the highest level of people

They are content. They know how to live or die. They have done something for society. They have reached the apex of life. They are eternal. For example: Lord Rama, Lord Krishna, Mahatma Gandhi, Jesus Christ, Swami Daynand, great warriors, and Prophet Mohammad; they are the greatest assets to the world. They will always be remembered. They are immortal.

Most people fall into categories two or three. People who get to level four have at least achieved their mission of life. But one who gets to level five becomes an asset to the world and/or human race.

Lessons that had helped me personally

I would like to share some of the lessons of my life that have helped me a great deal. They may or may not be applicable to you, but these are good insights and thoughts.

Everybody is okay.

We must understand that everybody tries their best. This is an important fact that needs due consideration. We need to understand that people behave differently because they have different education, different upbringing, different backgrounds, and different life experiences.

Every situation is okay.

One should never be surprised by any situation, even those that pop out of a blue moon, because there are so many variables.

We are just a number.

One of the biggest revelations of my life is the understanding that although we may believe that we are the most important persons, in reality and in the opinion of all others (equal to six billion people), we are just a number. This point needs serious concentration and can help a great deal.

A friendly atmosphere brings peace.

In the interest of everyone, it is important to create a friendly atmosphere everywhere, because it provides tranquility, peace of mind, and mental stability, not only for the others but also for the self.

Good words reap friendships.

A good kind and loving word can sow a seed of friendship.

Harsh words make enemies.

Equally, harsh and cruel words can make enemies.

It is a virtue to help others.
Helping others is one of the greatest virtues of any human being. Becoming good and becoming the best in oneself is not good enough. All of the greatest souls have had something to offer to others.

Nothing in life is wasted.
Nothing in this universe goes to waste. Every thought, every word, and every act will produce its effect or reaction. The effect of reaction can be immediate or delayed, so think twice before you say or do anything.

Follow a great role model.
One should choose one or more role models to follow in life for the purpose of transformation. It helps to create a framework.

Benefits

The first and the foremost step in transformation or for any change is your decision, without which nothing is possible. Once you have made a decision from your heart and soul, without any ifs or buts, half the battle is won. Now here is the process:

- Write the goals that you wish to accomplish. But the first and the foremost goal should be to live the life of health, happiness, and freedom, no matter what else you may want to achieve.

- Create a plan with a goal in mind. You may change the plan or the goal later if needed.

- Take the first step. All creation, all transformation, all long journeys, all achievements start with the first step.

- Analyze and watch your every step.

- Stay focused on the goal at all times.

Start your journey now

Your goal > create a plan > take the first step > analyze at every step > stay focused on the goal at all times. You will get there!

Key Message

Remember you are a magician, and you can create magic in your life. Think about it.

Mantra

I am in charge and a master of my life. I can create any change or transformation in my life, as long as I am willing, determined, and committed. I have the power to do whatever I wish to do.

CHAPTER THIRTY-THREE

Upbringing of the Children

One of the most important lessons that every child should learn is how to stay calm, collected, balanced, and happy in life; at least not to lose oneself in new and trying situations or negative outcomes of life. This is one of the fundamental secrets to a happy life.

Mentally calm, collected, balanced, and happy kids are the product of calm, collected, balanced, and happy parents. Do you agree? Two thumbs up to those parents who teach their children the value of the life and happiness. Happy kids and happy adults create a positive atmosphere everywhere, at home, in school, and in society. Healthy and happy children are in great need and demand for a healthy and happy nation and world.

Children are the future world. If we want a better future, better nation, and better world, then we need to place intense focus on the development, growth, education, and upbringing of our children. Whether our nation or world in the future will be a place of peace, rest, harmony or a place of unrest and disharmony will depend upon our children, and how they are raised and what they learn.

One can say that the upbringing of children is the responsibility of the parents. It is true to a great extent. But in reality it is everyone's responsibility, because we are all concerned for our future.

Some parents' expectations are quite nearsighted. They feel content if their children get a good education and good jobs and learn to take care of themselves and/or their parents in old age. It is too little to expect from a child. Of course children should take care of their parents as one of their moral and ethical duties. But equally important is the fact that children must learn to contribute to the well being of the nation and the world.

Objectives

From early on a child must learn:

Potential

Every child has huge potential. The sky is the limit. Children must be made aware that they can learn anything and can become anything.

Happiness

They must learn to stay happy in life. If they do not learn how to lead a healthy and happy life, than money, position, power, or anything else will be of a limited value.

Balance

They must learn how to maintain their balance in all the successes and failures of life. All these things are part of life. To run away or to commit suicide in the event of a negative outcome is the sign of failure.

Responsibility

They must learn that they will have the responsibility not only for themselves but also for all others, including parents, teachers, friends, relatives, and the community. However, if they want to go a step further, they should realize that they have responsibility towards the nation or even the world. They could make this world a better place.

Respect

In order to get respect they must respect all others. This is the only way.

Introduction

Children are the most important commodities we could ever have. Teaching children to live happily is as important as giving them good academic or vocational training. As parents we must teach our children very clearly that both success and failure are part of life, so that children don't give up, run away or commit suicide in the event of a negative outcome. It is sad and disheartening when you read or hear the stories of students committing suicide. Everyone feels like a failure.

The growth and development of a child is not an easy process. It is not the job of a single parent, teenage mother, or uneducated parents. One may need to use all the available resources. The role of uncles, aunts, and grandparents, teachers, and good-intentioned friends can be positive and immense. Although parents usually do everything in their power to give the best to their children, however, if they do not know how to give the proper guidance, then their children may not be the best. Upbringing is not merely feeding a child. It involves fostering mental and spiritual growth as well.

Children are very tender and innocent. So they need to be protected specially in their early years, from the wild life, selfish adults, or mean-natured people.

Education of children at home and school

Maharishi Swami Dayanand Saraswati in his book titled *Life of Truth* states:

> "Education plays a major role in the development of the child. To give the children the highest education and to instruct them in the way of truth, to make them refine in character and manners, in short to devote all their resources of body and

> mind, to accomplish this object is the paramount duty, the highest virtue, and the glory of the parents."

Children are wonderful. Their potential is huge. They can be made to learn anything and everything.

Values of life

Although schools are doing a good job in professional and vocational training; if children do not learn the values of life and do not learn how to deal with high and lows of life, then they will not be happy adults. If that is the case, then schools and parents cannot be considered doing good jobs.

Furthermore it is true that teachers feel less and less able to exercise authority over children. They are afraid to discipline kids without being blamed for abuse. This is sad. I'm not advising parents and teachers to use corporal punishment, but they must have the right to discipline children when they think it is appropriate.

Parents are equally to blame. They leave all the duty of education, mental and spiritual growth to the teachers. Teachers have their own limited role. With more and more being asked every day, teachers can do only so much. Also, moral, ethical, and spiritual values cannot be taught in school alone. These values must be learned at home first and then practiced at school; only then can they become part of child's life. This job cannot be done without the help of dedicated parents with whom the children spend sixteen hours a day. So teachers and parents need to become partners in the upbringing of healthy and happy children.

Ideal parents and ideal children

Fruit does not fall far from the tree. Ideal children come from ideal parents. If parents do not live an ideal life, then they should not expect anything better from their children. Children learn what they see and not just what they hear or are taught in words. If you study the history or the family background of alcoholics, drug addicts, and gamblers, you will be amazed to find that their parents were usually of the similar background. Conversely if you study ideal children, you will understand that these children also come from ideal parents. Inasmuch as children are the reflection of the parents, it is equally true that parents are also the reflection of their children.

In other words to have ideal children, parents have to become role models themselves; that is the only way, unless you know otherwise. Children learn what they live.

The role of sanskara in raising children and instilling values

Sanskara: What are these?

Sanskara means purification. The idea of sanskara is to communicate with the child and with the supreme. Sanskara are like the events in a religious or a conductive environment, when the message is conveyed to a child at nine different occasions before the age of five. There are seven more sanskara in additions to those nine. These are essential in the life of any individual. These sanskara help the child and the parents to become stronger and healthier. The information and knowledge provided in sanskara is for mental and spiritual development and is complementary to education that children receive in schools.

As you study the following sanskara, you will understand how deeply rooted the philosophy is in Vedas. How much both parents need to be involved jointly, physically, mentally, and spiritually in upbringing of their children. This in the long run pays big dividends.

These sanskara are gifts to the world from Swami Dayanand Saraswati of India. These sanskara guide us to how to inculcate moral, and ethical, and spiritual values. Maharishi Swami Dayanand Ji has taken this information from Vedas (book of knowledge) for the benefit of humanity.

How to raise children; how to teach the basic values; how to raise them into an ideal adults; how to teach them to respect their elders and not to be arrogant; how to teach them to be the best, yet not to give up in the face of calamities and/or failures of life; how to make a child welcome in the family even before conception; how to guide children to become part of the society and nation. These are some of the questions and issues that Swami Dayanand Ji discussed, in his book, *Light of Truth,* Chapter Two, Upbringing of the Children.

The essence of nine sanskara:

1) *Garbhadhan sanskara*: This is done on the day when both parents decide to have a baby, i.e., before conception. This sanskara affects the psychic and causal element (subconscious mind) of both parents, which in turn will influence the physic and causal elements (subconscious mind) of the conceived child. Parents pray to God, "Oh God! Our child should be great for the family, nation, and the world." (Behold, my friends, how positive thoughts, positive emotions, and positive feelings of the parents are aroused even before conception of the child. Can you imagine the expectations of the parents in the case of accidental pregnancy and/or rape?)

2) *Punsawan sanskara*: Two or three months after conception, this sanskara is performed. It is mainly meant to strengthen and purify the physical body of the conceived child. (Again observe how positive thoughts may affect the child while he is still in the womb!)

3) *Seemantorayan sanskara*: This sanskara is performed four to eight months after conception. This sanskara is meant to strengthen and purify the psychic and casual elements (subconscious mind) of the child still in the womb.

4) *Jakarta sanskara*: This sanskara is performed within a week of the birth of a child. The father or mother imprints God's name ("OM, God") on the tongue of the newly-born child.

5) *Namkaran sanskara*: This sanskara is performed when the child is 11 to 101 days old. Here the child is given a name based on the qualities that the parents desire in their child. The name given has to be meaningful and should represent the ideals that the parents wish in their child. Many parents give little or no importance in naming the child. If a child is given the name that has no meaning and or conveys no message, then how it could have any positive impact on the life of a child? (Hence before naming the child, the parents should give due and serious consideration and not just put a name tag (from A-Z) for the sake of identification.)

6) *Nishkaman sanskara*: Within three or four months of birth, the child should be taken to natural surroundings outside the home, and this sanskara should be performed to get the body and soul of the child attuned to the creation of God and nature.

7) *Annaprashan sanskara*: When a child is about six months old, light cereal food is given to them, and this sanskara is performed to draw attention to the necessity of purity and strength of the physical body. (Some parents start feeding their children too early, causing problem of allergies.)

8) *Choodakarma or Mundan sanskara*: With this sanskara, the child is given their first haircut when they are about a year old. This sanskara is meant for cleanliness and lessons of purity in their life.

9) *Karnavedha sanskara*: When a child is three to five years old, this sanskara is performed. Holes are made in the outer hanging or lower portions (lobes) of their ears. This is done to obviate them from certain ailments in life.

Do you appreciate the depth and philosophy of the sanskara?

Other issues in upbringing

Swami Ji has stressed the following issues in addition to the above mentioned sanskara:

1. *Brahamcharya*: Children should be kept away from sexual activities and attractions during their academic years. Keeping them away from sexual attractions helps them to devote all of their time to personal development and their studies.

2. Children should be kept at awe (disciplined). Parents should be firm but not too strict in raising their children, so that they may not become lazy. A definite line should be drawn between love and discipline. Parents who love immensely at the cost of discipline will spoil their children, and that can interfere with the mental and spiritual development of the child.

3. A child should learn the basic values of life, for example, respecting elders, not stealing, telling the truth, not being arrogant, having an attitude of gratefulness, speaking sweet language, and knowing the importance of a vegetarian diet.

4. Even in those days (120 years ago), Swami Ji mentioned that children should not be obese. He advised them not to overeat or at least never to eat to a full stomach, in keeping with Ayurvedic principles.

5. He also advised that if the mother cannot breast feed, cow's milk or goat's milk diluted 50-50 with water is nutritious.

6. He also mentioned that any dry food, for example, fried food and chips are not nutritious and should be avoided.

7. Swami Ji stressed the importance of proper pronunciation of the alphabet. It has an impact on the speech of the child.

8. Children should also learn to lead a balanced life, not to be upset with sorrows and not to be overjoyed with positive situations or outcomes. They should work hard to succeed, but not to get depressed or commit suicide in the event of crisis or failures. Children should be taught that successes and failures are part of everybody's life.

9. There should be constant desire for knowledge, control of senses, and the importance of good companionship.

10. Stories of the heroism, patriotism and of bhakta (devotion) should be part of a child's daily nighttime recital.

11. Children should be warned that they should stay away from deep water, unless advised by the teacher and the parents, because of dangerous animals, like crocodiles, could be present.

Practical points

Parents must understand:

- Need: Strong healthy and ideal children are needed not only for the family, but also for the nation and for the world.

- Happiness: It is the responsibility of the parents to make sure that children learn the basic values of life and happiness.

- Role model: The best way to teach a child is not by the words, but by action. This is the only way.

- Reflection: Inasmuch as children are the reflection of the parents, equally parents are also the reflection of their children.

- Duty: The parents' duty does not end with giving children a good education and making them independent. Parents must also make sure that their children learn the value of good health and happiness.

Little children usually think that their parents are almighty and know everything. When those children become teenagers they usually think that their parents know nothing, but when the teenagers become mature adults, they begin to realize the wisdom of their parents.

Warning/Caution

We must appreciate what our parents have done for us.

We all were children at one time. We owe much to our parents. They have done their best in raising us, based on their knowledge, experience, and resources. They could have been wrong at times but remember they did not have any formal training; it was hands-on experience. From being totally dependent, they have made us independent and have prepared us for this world. For that cause, they have utilized all the resources they had. Remember this: Respect your parents for what they have done. If you would have been in their place probably you would not have done much better. Furthermore, if you do not love, respect, and honor your parents, probably your children will treat you in a similar manner. They learn what they see and not so much by what you say.

Today maybe is the right time to call your parents, acknowledge, and thank them for what they have done for you. Even if they are dead, pray for their souls. It is a win-win situation. It will help your soul and theirs. It will also help your children to develop these qualities.

Mantra

I know parents and children are a reflection of each other. The best way I can teach anything to my children is by becoming a good role model. I also know that life is full of ups and downs; therefore, it is my paramount duty to teach the children how to stay calm and balanced under all situations and difficulties.

CHAPTER THIRTY-FOUR

One Universal Dharma/Religion: The Duty

What is the role of Dharma/religion in one's well being and happiness?

Dharma/religion guides us to the right duty, right path, and the right action. The right action means positive outcome. Positive outcome means a good and happier life.

Right duty →right action → positive outcome → happier life

In this chapter, we will not discuss dogmas, beliefs, rituals or even whether or not you should believe in religion (and/or God), because that is a personal matter, and everyone is free to make that decision. Instead, we will learn how Dharma/religion can act as a guiding light to the right path, right duty, and the right action. Schools and colleges do not teach Dharma/religion, although most parents do a fairly good job, but this cannot be said of all parents.

Vedas (the book of knowledge) has defined Dharma in two sentences:

1. Oh, man, do your duty!
2. Follow the right path.

You can read, recite, and appreciate the depth of these two small phrases. They are the nutshell of Dharma. This is the path of success and happiness. In this reference, I personally believe:

"If any great soul can show me the right path and guide me through the path, he will be my guru, mentor, and swami. I will owe my life to him. Such is the importance of Dharma, the duty, the path."

Objectives

1. The real purpose of Dharma/religion is to guide to righteousness of the duty of the individual.

2. A person who follows the right path is known to have good Dharma. It makes no difference whether one is Hindu, Christian, Muslim, Jewish, or anything else.

3. Dharma and religion are two different entities and hence need to be differentiated.

Introduction

Understanding your duty is a very basic necessity. Everybody has a duty to perform, whether they are a student, husband, wife, a top executive, or one at the bottom of the ladder in a corporation, or maybe a soldier on a battlefield. Life itself is a duty. Without fulfillment of your duty, your life could be miserable. The respect and honor given to you is based upon how well you perform your duty.

Definitions

1. According to *The Oxford Dictionary*, Dharma is defined as an Indian religion, eternal laws of cosmos, inherited in the very nature of the things. In Sanskrit, literature means decree or custom, whereas religion is defined as worship of a personal God, also a particular system of faith and worship.

   Dharma carries such a wide connotation that many people have defined it differently. Dharma is a guide to righteousness or to your call for duty.

2. One of the simplest definitions of Dharma is "to fulfill one's moral, ethical, and spiritual duties to the self and others." (Vedic view of life)

3. Another definition of Dharma is "the unprejudiced and the just way of living, e.g., truthfulness, kindness, compassion, and love for all."

4. Impartial justice, acceptance of truth, total abandonment of untruth, such conduct is Dharma, states Swami Dayanand Saraswati. (One of the greatest authorities on Vedas)

5. Sanatan Dharma is defined by Manusmriti in the following words: "Sanatan Dharma means always speak the truth. Speak the truth but not with bitterness. Speak with sweetness. Do not speak lies that are appealing."

6. According to Vedantic philosophy, Dharma is defined as "self-realization," i.e., understanding self.

7. "Kindness is Dharma, and ego is anti-Dharma," according to Kabir Das (one of the greatest poets of India).

From all the above definitions, you can appreciate that Dharma is something universal. It is based upon moral, ethical, and spiritual values, and has no connotation of religion or faith.

Dharma from religion, differentiation

Dharma and religion are two entities, although often confused or misinterpreted as one. Religion is defined as a cult, sect, or faith of certain group or class of people, whereas Dharma defines the attributes of the person without reference to religion or faith.

Religion: Why do people shun it?

1. Some people are not deeply into philosophy. To them life means eating, drinking, fun, and enjoyment. They believe that they have done their best if they have enjoyed life.

2. Some people were never exposed to religion because their parents were never into it.

3. Some people believe only those things that they can see with their eyes, hear with their ears, smell with their nose, and taste with their tongue, and so on. But the subject of religion is deep and abstract, hence not for them.

4. Some people erroneously believe that religion is just for priests, monks, and swamis.

5. Some people get turned away when they see fights and arguments in the religious places and temples. There has been a lot of blood shed in the past in the name of religion. Religion cannot be blamed for all this bloodshed. (It is the fault of a few religious leaders and not the religion itself. These religious leaders have exploited the public, either from their own misunderstanding of the religion or out of their own selfishness.)

6. Ego: Some people do not believe that religion is something more powerful than they are. They erroneously believe that they can control their own fate and the fate of the world. Some of the extreme examples are Alexander the Great, Hitler, King Hiranakasp, and King Karan.

All religions – Meta-analysis

All religions (not Dharma) can be studied in their four components:

1. God
2. Philosophy
3. Rituals
4. Spiritual values and universal virtues

These are the heart and soul of Dharma and/or religion.

<u>God</u>

The subject of God is discussed in Chapter 35 of this book. Remember one thing: even if you do not believe in God, you can still practice Dharma and/or be spiritual or good.

Philosophy

All religions have a different philosophy, but the philosophy of Dharma is universal. Philosophy is abstract and for an average individual that could be hard to understand. Interestingly it is important to know that one does not need to understand the philosophy of religion to become spiritual or good.

Rituals

Rituals vary from religion to religion, tribe to tribe, locality to locality, family to family, and even from person to person. Rituals create a religious and positive environment, but they are not important from a religious or spiritual point of view. At times rituals may have a negative effect. When one gets too obsessed with ritual, it can create fear and dependency that is against any religion. Religion is supposed to remove fear and provide mental and emotional strength and support.

Spiritual and universal virtues

Values and virtues are probably the most important aspects of Dharma and/or religion. To me, they are the heart and soul of Dharma and of all religions. The following couplet from the sixth chapter of the Manusmriti defines these virtues: *"Dhriti, kshama, damosteyam, Showchamindrya, nigrahah, hir vidya, satymakrodho, Dashakam lakshanam."*

Now the English translation of the above couplet: "Patience, forgiveness, self-control (control of the mind), honesty, and cleanliness, control of the senses, wisdom, knowledge, truth, and love are the ten characteristics of Dharma."

There is no religion that will argue against these virtues, and most religions do teach them. Do you know how many religions or people really practice this philosophy?

One universal religion

The question has come up in the past: Is it possible to combine all religions into one universal religion? Let us hear from Swami Vivekananda, an authority in this matter. He states:

> "It is not possible to put six billion people in one belief system. Quite often one cannot make even two people agree on one issue. But religion is such a broad subject; how could all of the people in the world agree unanimously on such a subject? If that would happen, there will be perfect balance, and perfect balance means all neutrality, which means inactivity and death. Variety is the first principle of life and unity lies in diversity. Electricity flows from positive to negative, not from positive to positive, not from negative to negative; water flows from high to low. If the ground is flat, water will get stagnant and will not flow. In every drama there has to be a hero and a villain (villen). This is the principle of action."

On the practical aspect, several attempts have been made in the history to unite all religions into a universal religion, and it has always failed, which is probably good. Swami Vivekanand believed that:

> "All religions lead to one God. As we get closer and closer to God, the difference between different religions gets less and less; so much so that when we reach the ultimate, there is no difference anymore. The further away we are from God, the more differences there are. Religion cannot be bad; God cannot be bad. We all need temples or churches. We all need religion. We need goodness. It is only a very tiny fraction of people who create the uproar or differences or even hatred in the name of the religion."

Dharma of humanity

This can be summarized in three words: compassion, kindness, and justice. Anyone who practices these virtues, in a real sense, practices the "Dharma of humanity," irrespective of being Christian, Hindu, Jewish, Muslim, or anything else.

Dharma/religion: method and means, not the goal

One needs to understand that the method and means (route and paths) are very different than the goal and/or the mission of anything. Here are two examples:

1. Let us say I want to get a BA or MA degree. Now going to college, paying hard-earned money for tuition, buying textbooks, studying hard for four years, and attending classes on daily basis are the method and means and not the goal. The goal will be to get a degree.

2. Now let us take another example; say I want to go to India from the U.S. The method and means will be to buy the plane ticket, pack the luggage, go to the airport, and catch the plane. But the goal is to reach India.

So it should be clear to everyone that Dharma/religion is the method and means and not the goal of life. The goal of life should be to become a good and kind person, and also to get rid of one's ego, so that one can enjoy the life of relaxation, health, and happiness.

Whether you believe in Krishna or Rama, Jesus Christ or Virgin Mary, Dayanand or Ganesha, Kali Devi or Lata Wali, Guru Nanak Dev or Mohammad or anyone else; it does not matter. What really matters is, will it help you to become a good person or not?

Some readers may not agree with me on this point, and they are welcome to their opinion. But since this is my opinion, I have taken the liberty to express it in my book.

Dharma and related subjects

- Religion and science
- Religion and politics
- Religion and spirituality

Religion and science

Religion and science are complementary. There should not be any confusion about it. The reason I want to open this issue for discussion is that at times naïve scientists and fanatical religious leaders clash on these issues.

Some scientists make slight of religion, and some religious leaders make slight of science. Science is based on logic, and religion is based on feelings and emotions. In science, feelings and emotions have no place, and in the religion, at times, there is no logic. Science provides technology and physical comfort; religion provides comfort to the soul and the mind.

Some religious people believe that scientists are fooling with the environment, and some scientists believe that religious leaders are fooling the lay people and deluding them with false hopes of salvation. I wish to assert here once again that science and religion are both essential and complementary to each other.

Religion and politics

Religion and politics are two different games of life. In religious places, politics has no role. Conversely in political associations or organizations, religion has no place. In any religious organization, if politics is going to prevail, it will cause the destruction of the organization; however when religion becomes part of the politics, politics may get a fine tune-up.

We must learn a great deal from the recent election of the Pope. I was amazed at the way the election took place. It was the most idealistic situation one could ever see. The election was conducted behind closed doors, no media, and no public involvement. The general public was kept out of sight. This was the best compromise between religion and politics.

Religion and politics - differences

Now let us try to analyze the differences between religion and politics:

1. In religion, one learns to respect and love others, but in politics one learns to outsmart and control others.

2. In religion, one learns to treat everyone equally, but in politics one tries to put others down.

3. In religion, one conquers one's internal enemies to find peace and happiness within the self. In politics, one tries to control other people to gain power and at times ends up in losing one's peace.

4. In religion, one learns to control one's ego, and in politics it is the game of ego.

5. Religion teaches the truth and nothing but the truth, and in politics truth hardly ever prevails.

6. In religion, there is no place for fights, but in politics fighting is commonplace.

7. In religion, one tries to find what is good and positive in others, but in politics one tries to find what is bad and negative in others to win the game.

8. A person of good Dharma would compromise and avoid arguments, whereas politicians love to argue.

Religion and spirituality

This was discussed in Chapter 22. Swami Agnivesh Ji said it beautifully: "What religion is to the individuals, spirituality is for the group."

Tests

Is your Dharma good?

As I mentioned before, Dharma and religion are two different entities. Religion defines the belief system or the philosophy of the sect of certain class of people, whereas Dharma defines the attributes of a person. If you are a good person, then your Dharma is good. However if you are bad, then your Dharma is bad. It has nothing to do with being Hindu, Muslim, Christian, Jewish, Sikh, or anything else.

What is a good person? A good person is one who is the owner of good thoughts, words, and actions. If you would like to differentiate good from bad, see the chapter on spirituality (Chapter 22).

Is your religion good?
To my understanding, religion means something good. It is supposed to make a person good or better. However if a person has not benefited from their religion, it reflects only the ignorant side of the person, and not of the religion. Therefore religion of that person cannot be discredited.

What is your Dharma/what are your duties?
Can you sincerely and honestly talk to yourself about what kind of person you are, what principles you live by, how you make your decisions? Are you conscious and aware of your duties?

Try to analyze your duties:
1. Towards yourself
2. Towards others
3. Towards your country
4. Towards humanity
5. Towards God (if you believe in God)

Your attributes and characteristics define your Dharma. It has no direct relationship with the religion you embrace.

The key message
Dharma is only one, although there are many religions. Dharma defines the attributes of the person. Dharma is the religion of humanity. If you breed love, kindness, compassion, and acceptance of all others, you are known to be a person of good Dharma. It matters little whether you are

Hindu, Christian, Muslim, Jewish, or anything else. As a matter of fact, in order to possess those qualities you do not have to belong to any religion.

The second part of the definition of Dharma is that if you do your duty right, irrespective of the result, you are also known to be a person of good Dharma. Lord Krishna use to say “Do your duty and do not worry about the reward.”

Mantra

I will constantly strive to become a just, kind and compassionate person. I will love all human beings. This is my Dharma. This is my duty.

CHAPTER THIRTY-FIVE

One Universal God: Concept of God

Let us begin this unique and abstract subject with two questions:

1. Is belief in God essential for health and happiness?
2. What is meant by the concept of God?

My understanding and observation is that people who sincerely believe in God from their heart and soul are generally healthier and happier than those who do not. Of course there are plenty of exceptions.

Coming to the second question, what is meant by the concept of God? After reading scriptures, I have come to the understanding that the words "good" and "God" are very much related, connected, and interwoven. As a matter of fact, the word "God" is derived from the word "good" by taking off one "o."

Furthermore we all understand that "God" or "goodness" is the basis of creation and sustenance of each and everything, whether it is an object, organization, government, or even a person. Conversely evil is the cause of dissolution of anything. This is what I meant about the concept of God. Whether you believe in God or the concept of God is your choice, but becoming a good or better person does contribute towards health and happiness.

There are a lot of honest, kind, and good people out there who do not believe in God, and I do respect them equally. And you may be one of them.

Objectives

1. Understanding God and/or the concept of God
2. How to benefit from the concept, even if one doesn't believe in God

Introduction

Who is He?

In the universe, energy is the basis of all creation, including you, me, and everything else. God is also energy. Therefore there is a hierarchy of energy. The whole universe is based on the cause and effect phenomenon. According to the cause and effect phenomenon, the higher or subtler level of energy is the cause, and the lower level of energy is the effect, and not vice versa. Since God is the subtlest of all, hence He is the cause of all creation.

Let us review briefly other examples of the cause and effect phenomenon. For example, dynamic energy is the cause, and an atom is the effect, because dynamic energy is subtler than an atom. Similarly an atom is the cause, and matter is the effect; here an atom is subtler than the matter. Also, the soul is the cause, and body is the effect, because the soul is subtler than the body.

Definition

God is very abstract. People define God differently according to their own perception and beliefs. People define the way they get their own solace, comfort, joy, and peace.

Swami Dayanand Saraswati, a spiritual monk of highest caliber, has defined God in the second principle of Arya Samaj as follows:

> "God is personification of existence, intelligence, and bliss. He is the creator, sustainer, and desolator. He is formless, almighty, just, benevolent, unborn, endless, and infinite. Unchangeable, beginning less, incomparable, support of all, and lord of all, all pervading, omniscient, controller of all from within, undeceiving, imperishable, fearless, eternal, and holy and maker of the universe."

Let me give you a little more insight into the word "God." Everything and anything that exists in nature is based on goodness. As soon as evil and negativity take over anything, i.e., a unit, organizations or life, that thing vanishes. Evil is the signal that it is time to perish. Or we can say God is good, and good is God.

If you analyze it further, the word God has three letters: G, O, D. Here **G** here stands for generator or creator, **O** stands for operator or sustainer, and **D** stands for desolator.

God and super-consciousness

According to Vedic principles, everything in this universe can be classified according to the level of consciousness:

Minerals – unconsciousness
Plants – level of consciousness between minerals and animals
Animals – lower level of consciousness
Human beings – higher level of consciousness
God – super-consciousness and hence blissfulness

Diverse views about God

Let us analyze some of the diverse views, about God:

<u>Perception</u>

Some people perceive Him sitting far, far away in heaven, while others believe that He is present in each and every place, including our heart and soul.

Faith

Some people die in His name; others think that people who believe in God are crazy.

His work

Some believe that anything and everything that happens is under His guidance and direction, whereas others believe it is all imagination and delusion.

Fear

Some people are afraid of Him, while others are not even afraid of cursing and blaming Him for each and everything bad that happens.

Fact/Fiction

Some people believe they were created by God; others believe that God is the creation of mankind.

Mystery

Most people do remember Him one time or another, usually when they are in pain/or when something mysterious happens. Maybe that's why He is a mystery.

Does God exist?

We tend to believe that if something is created, there has to be a creator. Nothing is created by itself. For example, a pen, a pencil, paper, and such are manufactured by a factory. Food is grown by farmers. Anything new is created by architects, and so on. Furthermore we live in this huge universe. It is so huge that the scientists of today have not been able to come up with the dimensions. Not only this, but our huge universe runs so smoothly and perfectly that it is mind-boggling. This has been going on for eternity. Who could be the creator of such a universe? Just wonder!

Just for thought: When I am alone!

There comes a time in everyone's life when you feel alone. You don't have anyone to speak to, anyone to share with, when your brothers and sisters are gone. Relatives live far away. Children are too busy. Friends are not available. You wish your parents were still alive. Then you realize that there is still someone you can speak with, someone who is willing to listen, someone you can share with, and that is Him.

Do I have to believe in God?

Whether you believe in Him or not, that is your choice. It is a question of your beliefs. If you want to believe only what you see with your eyes, what you hear with your ears, and what you feel with your hand, then you would not believe in Him. In the universe, things exist at the physical level, energy level, and super-energy level. Things that we see with our eyes are only those things that exist at the physical level. We do not see those things that exist at the energy and super-energy levels. For that, you need intuition and wisdom.

Do you see air? No, but you know and feel the power of the air. How long can you live without it? Just think. Do you see light, magnetism, electricity, or sound? No! However, you see the effect of these energies, but not the energy per se. If I ask you how electricity looks, you would not be able to define it in its physical form. If I ask you how sound looks, you would not be able to define it. If I ask you for the shape of magnetism, you would not be able to define it, either. Because these are energies, and energies have no size or shape. Similarly, God is energy/super-energy without any shape or dimensions.

You have not seen happiness, but you crave it. You cannot see love. You cannot see friendship. But you can feel the happiness, love, and friendship. Life would be miserable and painful without them.

We cannot depend just on our eyes for the sake of perception. We need all of our faculties to perceive things, e.g., hearing, smelling, touch, feeling, imagination, intuition, wisdom, and so on. And these are all complementary to each other for the purpose of perception.

You must have also noted whenever you are in trouble, helpless or lost spiritually, you say: "Oh, my Lord, oh, my God." How and from where do these words come? There must be some truth behind them.

I will tell you one thing emphatically that if you do not believe in God, you are not alone in this universe.

You must have observed that there are families in which the child and father don't get along. These are broken families. It is because of ignorance. But this is the way the world goes. Everybody lives with their own decisions and choices.

It is also my observation that people who believe in God with sincerity, love, and kindness also become kindhearted. Kindheartedness in itself is a virtue that makes them calm and brings them to the spiritual level. Spirituality makes them mentally and spiritually strong, and that, in turn, brings freedom and joy.

I sincerely believe that God doesn't punish anyone, even those who do not believe in Him. Just like if you don't love and respect your father or mother, they will not punish you. But you are setting an example for your own children as to how to treat parents. Caution! Be ready for it.

The concept of one universal God

God is one, not two, not three or four. This is based on at least two hypotheses. First, if there were two Gods, three Gods, four Gods, there could be a fight between the Gods maybe once in a million years, which could lead to disaster. Second, every religion teaches us that God is our father. In other words, my relationship with Him is that of a father and son.

We have also seen that some people change their religion for whatever reason. For example, some Hindus or Muslims become Christian or equally some Christians become Muslim, Hindu, and so on. If a Christian becomes Hindu, does it means that he has to divorce his Christian father and adopt the Hindu father, and vice versa? Is it possible to change one's father?

It is true that most religions (not all) believe in their own messenger which is unique to that religion. Could we say that all of these messengers were children of only one God? All of these messengers have brought a good message to the humanity in a time of need in a different way. But unfortunately at times, the message is misinterpreted or misunderstood.

Real life example: An interesting story

Have you ever seen two children fighting with each other about their mother, each one says she is my mom and she loves me very much. This happens in front of the mother, and she just laughs. When the first child asks his mother, "You are my mom and you love me very much, don't you?" She replies, "Yes, of course, I love you very much." And the child feels secure. Now the second child asks the same question to her mother, and she again laughs. She repeats the same answer "Yes, of course, I love you very much." This is the story of ignorant people fighting about one God.

How we are connected with God

Relationship with God

He is related to me as my father. Whatever relation I have with my children, I have similar relationship with Him. I care for my children very dearly; so does He. I love my children very much; so does He. I want my children to be happy, healthy, and prosperous; so does He. I believe my biggest gift to my children is education; so does He. So God has given all knowledge to the mankind in the form of Vedas, the Bible, and other scriptures. Different messengers of different religions have put forth the information in their own version and that information came from God. I believe that if all these messengers were to appear again I am sure they would not or could not discriminate, whether one is Hindu, Christian, Muslim, or Jewish or anything else.

Where does He live?

He lives with me, as I live with my children, in the same city and same house, same room, and same body. If He would live away from me in a different town or different city or different state or different planet, then He could not be my father. As He is the father of the universe, He has to be everywhere. In order to be present everywhere, He has thinned out Himself in the form of super-energy to become omnipresent.

God as a provider

God provides us with each and every thing. All good things are free. There is free air, free water (spring water), and free land (unless you live in a sophisticated house). Your vision, hearing, smell, taste, touch, and your body are all free. Joy, laughter, and happiness are all free. There is also free intelligence, wisdom, joy, or the will to act; even this life is free. Look at wildlife, sea life, underdeveloped countries: do they pay for all these necessities of life? Also look at the homeless people living in the U.S., one of the richest countries of the world; they don't pay for anything. We pay because we are civilized and too sophisticated.

Who is the victim?

One may be surprised with this title but I am not! I observe all the time that people often blame God for all the pain and suffering of theirs and the world's. This is true of not only some people who believe in God, but also of people who do not believe in God. As a matter of fact, this is one of the explanations given by some of the people as to why they do not believe in God. They often say if there is God, then why there is so much pain, suffering, and misery? As if God is the cause of all the bad things in life. And people who do believe in God at times also think that pain and miseries is due to the fact that God is angry.

God by definition is just. We are rewarded or punished for our own deeds by the universals laws of nature and not by Him. Neither He punishes, nor, He likes to punish! Now tell me who is the victim, you, or God?

God and fear

It is amazing how the word fear is attached to God, sometimes in a positive way and others in a negative manner. You know some people will not commit a wrong act because of their fear of God. Others will not hesitate to commit a wrong act because they believe that God will forgive them.

How He runs the universe

What does He do?

This question should rather be phrased as, what He does not do. He does everything, He creates, sustains, or maintains everything, and when things become evil, bad, and useless He desolates. He also has an influence on everything that has a lower frequency, and that means everything. This is exactly what we do in our homes (later on in this chapter).

Universal laws

He runs His universe through these laws that do not change for anyone, because He loves everyone, and He is just.

Automation

Everything is automated in His universe: birth, death, punishment, reward, creations, and dissolution. He does not reward or punish day to day, case by case, or person by person, but according to universal laws which are automated like a computer. We all have a chip built into our subconscious mind which monitors all of our activities, good and bad, positive and negative. Accordingly we get rewarded or punished by the universal laws of nature. This is how God keeps tabs on us.

Motion

Everything in the universe is energy. And energy by definition cannot stay still, so everything is in motion. It is amazing to see that in the universe everything is in motion, and very rapid motion, yet there is no noise. It is hard to comprehend, because according to our observation whenever something moves it creates friction and noise. But everything in this universe moves at unimaginable speed, yet we hear no noise. For example, Earth is moving 1.8 million miles per day. I'm sure there are things moving much faster rate than this speed, yet it is all calm, all quiet, and all noiseless. It is an art and beauty of the creator and creation. Do you know how, because in the universe things are moving in empty space? There is no matter; it is all empty, so there is no friction and no noise. What a beauty! If the Earth's motion would create noise, we would go crazy.

Nothing goes to waste. Everything is recycled.

Nothing goes to waste in this universe, not even an atom or an electron. Everything is recycled again and again. Even our body is recycled. This can be explained on the basis that energy is the foundation of all creations, and energy cannot be destroyed by any definition.

There are two types of energy, namely dynamic and static. Dynamic energy can be transformed into static energy, i.e., the physical form. Also physical form (static energy) can be changed into dynamic energy. So dynamic energy and physical form are interchangeable. The physical form is just the condensed form of dynamic energy.

Once energy gets condensed, it gets fixed, becomes less powerful, less available. There are several types of energy: light, heat, sound, electricity, and magnetism, and all of them are interchangeable from one form to another. For example, heat can be changed into electricity; electricity can be changed into heat. Electricity can be changed into magnetism, and vice versa. Similarly sound can be changed into electricity, magnetism or heat etc.

Why things are cyclical in nature: to avoid waste

In this universe everything is cyclical in nature. One cycle means something leaves its home, does its job, and then goes back to its home. This is one cycle. For example, the home of the water is the ocean. It leaves the ocean, makes the clouds, and rains. Now it goes back to the ocean.

Similarly the home of fire is the sun. With the heat of the sun, food and wood grows. When wood burns it makes fire. The fire goes up as it is attracted to the sun. The reason being the house of fire or heat is the sun. Now take the example of air. The house of air is atmosphere. We breathe in air and liberate carbon dioxide. This air goes back to the atmosphere, its home. Similarly we come from God and go back to Him.

Everything must go home to continue the cycle over and over again. This is how water, air, nitrogen, life, and anything that is cyclical in nature behaves and works. This is the principle of recycling.

Laws of creation

God creates things when the need arises. He maintains them as long as they are useful and beneficial, and when things become useless and evil, He destroys them. It is exactly what we do. We bring home good things when we need them. We maintain them as long as they are useful, and when these become useless or broken, we destroy them or throw them away.

In the universe everything is for the benefit of mankind.

There is nothing in the universe that is not useful. Maybe we do not understand with our little imagination and understanding. For example, snakes are anti-pollution; they are the best friends of the farmer because they kill rats. Rats are good friends of the farmer because they soften the land, and so on. There are many more similar examples.

His teaching

Vedas states: O man rise, and become noble. O men make the world noble.

Just behold what is expected of us. The word "noble" means excellent. Noble is beyond good and very good. Nobleness does not come until one extends beyond oneself in the form of love, compassion, sacrifice or devotion. No matter how good people may be, they may not eat meat, drink alcohol, or smoke; they may never have lied or stolen, but that does not make them noble or divine.

The word "divine" means superb, excellent, and God-like. Unless one becomes divine, one will not find happiness, bliss, and salvation. Eternal happiness and bliss have a basis on goodness, nobleness and divinity.

In search of GOD

How we can find God?

"Seek and you shall find Him." If you have intense desire for anything, you will find it. If you have intense desire for Him, you will find Him. But you have to become like Him to perceive Him. This is natural. You see, when you go to a temple you dress with simple and clean clothes. When you go to a dance, you dress with fancy and elegant clothes. When you go to karate class, you dress with sporty clothes so that you are able to perform as a karate student. You go to school and you dress in school clothes with a book bag.

Similarly when you need to perceive God, you have to come to His energy level, the spiritual level, the goodness level. But most people live only at the physical level. Because God does not exist at the physical level, it is very hard to perceive Him at that level.

To get to His energy, spiritual, and goodness level, you have to become good and spiritual. It is only then that you can perceive the joy of Him. You start appreciating Him, His creation, and His wisdom. Once you start appreciating His perfection, His vastness, His energy, and His love, you find peace, happiness, and blissfulness in your heart. This is the feeling of being with God.

The day you start to see everything as God's creation, the day you start to love everything and every being in this universe, you will find Him. No need to search anymore.

Prayer

Prayer is another way to find God. Prayer brings purification and self-realization, and it brings us closer to God. Some people believe that the purpose of prayer is to please God; that is not the case. He does not need to be pleased; He is always happy and blissful. As a matter of fact, it is very hard to displease him.

Let us see how prayer impacts our life even if we do not believe in God and how it can brings us closer to God. Prayer has several components and each has its own purpose.

<u>To praise God or count His attributes</u>

The idea of counting His attributes is to inculcate those qualities in our life.

<u>To sit with Him, to meditate on Him</u>

So that we can feel His strength, wisdom, depth, vastness, energy, and lastly and most importantly His love

<u>To ask for something</u>

When you are going to ask something of God, ask for the best things in life. Don't ask for little things. He is a big provider, so ask Him for big things. It is sad when people ask for little things, i.e., money, home, job. Vedas says intelligence is the highest gift to mankind, so why not ask for intelligence? You all know the importance and value of intelligence. It is the solution to all problems of life, and hence the cause of all happiness.

To thank Him for His provisions: This is also the time to connect with Him in appreciation. This makes you content, and that is a reward in itself.

To enter a positive mode
Our mind is wandering. It has to think about something, whether good or bad, right or wrong. Prayer is the time when our mind comes under focus and in a positive thinking mode. The more we pray, the more time we spend in a positive thinking mode.

To improve concentration
During the time of prayer we are connecting with supreme energy, the source of all energy, happiness, and bliss.

To have family prayer
There is an aphorism that states "The family that prays together stays together." Family prayer gives you a positive feeling and bonding with family members.

To partake in community/joint prayers in temples/churches
This has similar such multiple advantages.

Benefits of prayer for everyone: whether or not you believe in God
During prayer you are connecting yourself with your own heart and soul, even if you do not believe in God. Now try to recite or read the following mantra every day for one month without failure and see how it affects you.

Let me be strong.
Let me stay on the right path.
Let me love my neighbor.
Let me control my anger.
Let me be calm in all situations.
Let my intellect be keen.

You will appreciate the positive effects of this prayer on your mind and subconscious mind, irrespective of your belief in God, so prayer is for everybody.

The qualities and attributes of a God-realized soul

Let us see the qualities of the people who are God-realized souls and self-realized souls. God-realized souls are slightly different from the people who are self-realized souls.

Attributes of the self-realized soul:

- One realizes that they are the eternal soul, not the body or mind.
- One starts to realize the temporary nature of everything and anything, which includes money, position, power, family, and even their body.
- One starts to feel satisfied and content.
- As a result, one finds peace within the self.

Attributes of the God-realized soul:

- He sees everything as His creation.
- He accepts everything as it is, and does not criticize.
- He sees every living being as part of His family.
- He starts to understand and accepts the people who breed anger, hate, jealousy, and/or greed, as being innocent.
- He becomes kind, caring, loving, and compassionate.
- He sees God as the source of all bliss and love.
- He becomes blissful and emanates peace for self and others.

Benefits

Now let us see how everybody can benefit from this chapter, even one who does not believe in God:

For people who don't believe in God

Role model: According to this concept, God is defined as the personification of perfection and/or goodness. Perfection and/or goodness bring strength at all levels, including physical, mental, and spiritual. Strength brings freedom, and freedom brings happiness.

For people who believe in God

God is the source of all peace, joy, and bliss. Death is the most feared thing in life. Knowing that eventually we go with Him, gives us comfort. Also whenever a bad thought comes to mind, we quite often stop from wrongdoing for fear of being punished. Faith in God also builds faith in the self, because we know that God is with us at all times.

Neutral plan

Focus on any one property of God or any good quality of a person. Do this the first thing in the morning in your daily prayer. For example, think of love, kindness, compassion, truthfulness, sincerity, friendship, humility, gentleness, strength, or purity, and so on. Now stay focused on that quality for that day. If you do that on a regular basis, that quality will become part of your life and will help you to become a better person.

The key message

If you do not believe in God, then you could believe in the concept of God, i.e., becoming a kind and good person. However, if you believe in God, probably the best way to get closer to Him is to help your fellow beings. Remember your whole life is based upon helping others, whether it is at the level of family, social life, or even business life.

Mantra

I will believe either in God or in just becoming "good" (a kind person), because being a "good" (kind) person is the best and surest way to get closer to God and/or find joy and happiness in life.

Oh God, grant me the wisdom,
So that I can enjoy the life of happiness and freedom

Oh my God, grant me the wisdom
So that I can enjoy the life of happiness and freedom

Who could be as powerful as you?
Who could equal you?
If there could be another one like you
I fear to imagine, if there could be fight between the two
What could happen to this world?
Or what could happen to both of you

I understand pain and misery are part of life
As are bad and good times
Just like the summer and winter, or day and night
As are hero and villain, of each game
Whether I choose to play hero or villain
It is all up to me and my game
So how could you be ever blamed?
When I am choosing the role to play

We appreciate the messenger you send
At different times
Rama, Krishna, Jesus, and Mohammad, they
were all good and kind.
Please send some new ones
Because we are the desperate ones
To make us understand that we are all one
And you are the only father
Hindu, Muslim, Christian or all brothers
Most people fight out of confusion
If someone could remove that confusion,
Life would be much more joyful and fun

Every religion believes in their God (father)
Om, God, Allah are the multiple names of you
All religions also merge into you
When people change their religion
How can they change their Father?
Oh Lord, give us the power to understand the true effect
You are the only one, mighty and perfect

Call me Brother, Singhal or Pratap
Take my sincere advice
This life is an opportunity to become good or perfect
Goodness brings happiness and freedom
That should be everybody's mission
When one completes one's mission
When one treats everybody as a brother or sister
One merges into God, and God merges into one
So one enjoys the life of happiness and freedom

Oh Lord, it is my humble prayer
Grant us the wisdom
So we can enjoy the life of happiness and freedom

What to fear and whom to fear...
God is with me
I am with Him
Then what to fear
And whom to fear

Air, water, fire and the plants
Animals and human beings are His creation
Love of all is His only plan
Then what to fear
And whom to fear

No need to blame or fear God
He is only a helping hand
He could not hurt His own child
It is one of the secrets of life.
Then what to fear
And whom to fear

Everybody tells me He is our father
So He must have touched me with His hands
He must have kissed me with His lips
He must have embraced me closer to His chest
He must have loved me with all His heart
Then what to fear
And whom to fear

Oh God, you are the creator of this huge universe
And also of me
You are out there, and also in me
You are within me, and outside of me
Then what to fear
And whom to fear

SECTION IV

Doctor, I am Sick!

When one is afflicted with a disease or sickness, several questions come to mind. How did I get sick? What treatment options do I have? Can I be cured? The last question becomes important especially when one is afflicted with a chronic (lasting) disease.

There are several treatment options available to everyone, and all are unique. Every treatment modality has its own advantages and limitations. The superiority of the choice can be judged only by the patient based upon their knowledge, expectations, and needs. Although it is not possible to discuss all treatment options, I will discuss the most common ones. This should help you a great deal in making better treatment selections. It is best that all treatment modalities be considered complementary to each other.

I would also like to stress a very important fact: that true healing or cure happens only when one is 100 percent willing, determined, and committed. No doctor, hospital or any art of healing can replace this most important ingredient.

CHAPTER THIRTY-SIX

Conventional Medicine (Allopathy)

Conventional medicine is also known as modern or allopathic medicine. It is the medical science in vogue especially in the western world or for the people who want quick results. Like any other medical science, it has its limitations. One of the main reasons for the limitations of most healing medical sciences is that our body is very complex and is under the control of our mind or psyche. And our mind or psyche is not easily influenced by most drugs or medicines.

Objective

We need to broaden our horizons and open our mind and eyes to what else is available for our benefit.

Evolution

Everything evolves out of necessity; modern science is no exception. As man became smarter and smarter, he started to look for solutions to meet his medical needs, and medical sciences continued to evolve over centuries. Initially all healing sciences were one. It was later that it started to differentiate into conventional medicine or allopathy, natural medicine, Ayurveda, homeopathy, and so on. No doubt allopathy has made great advances in the field of emergency medicine, trauma, and surgery, but it can fall short when it comes to true healing.

Definition

Healing is defined as making one spiritually whole or complete. There is no such word as whole or spiritually whole in conventional medicine.

Philosophy

Allopathic medicine is based on the "law of contraries," i.e., opposites cure opposites. It is the exact opposite of the homeopathic philosophy which is based on the "law of similar."

In the law of contraries or the law of opposites, the patient is treated with the opposite modality, e.g., if the patient is hot, he is cooled and if he is cold, he is made warm. Similarly if the blood pressure is high, we bring it down, and if it is low, we bring it up, and so on.

Limitations

Limitations of allopathic medical science:

- It does not cure any chronic condition. However it is quite effective in relieving and or palliating the suffering.

- Every drug used in allopathic medicine has side effects, and at time these can be quite serious.

Benefits

Conventional medicine has many advantages. In emergency situations or trauma, there is no replacement to allopathic approach. Here doctors are true heroes. Diagnosis is quick, and the results are immediate.

CHAPTER THIRTY-SEVEN

Ayurveda & Maharishi Ayurveda: Healing at the Level of the Body, Mind & Soul

If you are searching for a medical science that can heal the person at all the three levels of your existence: body, mind, and soul, then probably it is Maharishi Ayurveda, at least to the best of my knowledge. Having said that, let us understand the origin and history of Ayurveda. The word Ayurveda comes from Sanskrit. *Ayur* means life, and *veda* means science.

Ayurveda and Maharishi Ayurveda are related medical sciences with some differences. Ayurveda is the oldest medical science that deals with health at the physical level, whereas Maharishi Ayurveda deals with health at the physical, mental, and spiritual levels. Ayurvedic medical science dates back 5,000 years, but the Maharishi Ayurveda is a relatively new science that evolved approximately 40 years ago, after his holiness, Mahesh Yogi, held a world health conference of all Ayurvedic physicians of the world in Bombay, India in 1968.

You should also differentiate Ayurveda from homeopathy.

Objectives

1. Understanding health in totality and completeness

2. Understanding how easy it is to use diet as a medicine, once you understand your constitution or Dosha type

3. Application of treatment modalities for strengthening the mind and the spirit that include meditation, sound, and so on

Introduction

Ayurveda is the oldest yet most comprehensive existing healthcare system; it originated in India from the ancient Vedic civilization. Ayurveda is translated as "science of lifespan." It is strongly oriented not only towards prevention of diseases but also towards maintenance of health and treatment of the diseases. Ayurveda has its roots in Vedas. (*Rig Veda* is the first book ever introduced into the Library of Congress).

Philosophy of Ayurveda

According to Ayurveda, our body is autonomous or self-governing, self-diagnosing, and self-regulating; i.e., our body is capable of self-diagnosing and then self-healing, which is a function of the intelligence of the body.

Definition of health: Ayurvedic perspective

The Ayurvedic definition of health is probably the most precise and complete definition that one will ever find. It covers all three aspects of health: physical, mental, and spiritual. Just behold the definition that follows: *Samadoshah samagnish ca samadhatumalakriyah prasannatmendriyamanah svastha ity abhidhiyate (Sushruta Sutrasthanam)***.** Translation: He whose Doshas are in balance, whose appetite is good, whose Dhatus are functioning normally, whose Malas are in balance, and whose self, mind, and senses remain full of bliss is called a healthy person.

Let us analyze this definition. Remember there are seven different components at the physical, mental, and spiritual levels.

Physical level

1. Doshas should be in balance. There are three Doshas, namely Vata, Pitta, and Kapha. I shall discuss these in details.

2. Dhatus should be functioning normally. Dhatu is the first gross physical structure formation, e.g., cells, tissues.

3. Malas should be in balance. These are the substances that are partly utilized and partly excreted. (These three elements Doshas, Dhatu, and Malas are said to be in dynamic equilibrium with each other for the maintenance of good health.)

4. Appetite must be good. Appetite according to Ayurveda is one of the most important functions of the body, because all the physical energy is gained through food.

5. All senses (eyes, ear, nose, tongue, skin) should be healthy.

6. Mind should be balanced.

7. Self or spiritual level: one should be content and blissful.

Concept of Doshas (constitution)

According to Ayurveda, the imbalance in physiology is known as Doshas. These Doshas have their origin in Pancha (five) Mahabhutas. Therefore let us understand these Mahabhutas first.

Pancha Mahabhutas

There are five Mahabhutas translated into English as *akasha* (sky), *vayu* (air), *agni* (fire), *jala* (water), and *prithvi* (earth). Although these five Mahabhutas may appear simple in English, they do not connote the correct and full implications of these words. For example, ordinary water does not contain Jala Mahabhutas alone but is composed of all five Mahabhutas. It is the force of cohesion or the power of attraction that is inherent in Jala (water). You all know that the water is made of oxygen and hydrogen; here oxygen is nearer to Agni Mahabhutas, and hydrogen nearer to Jala Mahabhutas. Similarly other four Mahabhutas: *vayu* (air), *agni* (fire), *prithvi* (earth) and *akasha* (sky) also have elements of other Mahabhutas.

Tridosha concept

There are three main types of Doshas: Vata, Pitta, and Kapha. These Doshas are based upon the imbalances in five Mahabhutas. The nearest English equivalents to these terms are Vata (air), Pitta (bile), and Kapha (phlegm). All three Doshas have the five Mahabhutas in their composition but in different proportions. In Pitta or Agni Dosha, the fire Mahabhuta is predominant. In Kapha Dosha, the water Jala and earth prithvi Mahabhutas are predominant. In Vata or Vayu Dosha, vayu the air Mahabhuta is predominant.

The Dosha as a conceptual phenomenon: This applies equally to the body humors, food, age, season, time of the day, etc. Let us understand in little details how it applies in life:

<u>Age</u>

Old age corresponds to Vata.
Youth corresponds to Pitta.
Child infancy and childhood corresponds to Kapha.

<u>Seasons</u>

Winter corresponds to Vata.
Summer corresponds to Pitta.
Spring correspond to Kapha.

<u>Time of the day</u>

Vata corresponds from 2:00 to 6:00 a.m. and from 2:00 to 6:00 p.m.

Pitta corresponds from 10:00 a.m. to 2:00 p.m. and from 10:00 p.m. to 2:00 a.m.
Kapha corresponds from 6:00 to 10:00 a.m. and from 6:00 to 10:00 p.m.

Food
Vata food is cold and dry.
Pitta food is hot and pungent.
Kapha food is rich, heavy, and sweet.

Dosha types: practical application to the body

Everybody should try to determine their imbalance or Dosha type and thereafter eat accordingly to correct that imbalance from which they may be suffering.

Although there are three main Dosha types: Vata, Pitta, and Kapha, however, these Doshas can exist in various combinations, e.g.: Vata and Kapha, Vata and Pitta, Pitta and Kapha, and so on. Whenever any Dosha goes out of balance, diseases start. During sickness a person may have an imbalance of one, two, or all three Doshas.

Following is a list of all of the classifications of different Dosha types. You can read and analyze how they apply to your body system. It may help you decide which type of predominant Dosha imbalance you have.

Characteristics of Vata type
1) Has lighter, thinner build, 2) performs activity quickly, 3) tends toward dry skin, 4) has aversion to cold weather, 5) has irregular hunger and digestion, 6) is quick to grasp new information, also quick to forget, 7) tends to worry, 8) tends to be constipated, 9) tends to have light and interrupted sleep.

Characteristics of Pitta type
1) Has moderate build, 2) performs activity with medium speed 3) averse to hot weather, 4) prefers cold food and drinks, 5) has sharp hunger and

digestion, 6) can't skip meals, 7) takes medium time to grasp new information, 8) has medium memory, 9) tends toward reddish hair and complexion, moles, and freckles, 10) is good at public speaking, 11) tends toward irritability and anger, 12) is enterprising and sharp in character.

Characteristics of Kapha type
1) Has solid, heavier build, 2) has greater strength and endurance, 3) is slow, methodical in activity, 4) has oily, smooth skin, 5) has slow digestion, mild hunger, 6) has tranquil, steady personality, 7) is slow to grasp new information, slow to forget, 8) is slow to become excited or irritated, 9) sleeps heavy and long, 10) has plentiful, thick, and wavy hair.

Maharishi Ayurveda for health and happiness

Ayurveda has a wider range of application in the prevention and treatment of diseases, because it offers help at the physical, mental, and spiritual levels. Let us discuss these under following subheadings:

A. Different modalities of treatment
B. How diets can help in balancing Doshas
C. Guidelines for proper digestion
D. Constipation

Different modalities of treatment in Ayurveda

Health is a very complex subject. To cover all aspects of health, many different modalities of treatments may be required. According to Maharishi Ayurveda, there are twenty such approaches, as follows:

1. Consciousness
2. Primordial sound
3. Intellect
4. Emotions
5. Language

6. Gandharv Veda
7. Sense
8. Pulse diagnosis
9. Psycho-physiological integration
10. Neuromuscular integration
11. Neuro-respiratory integration
12. Physiological purification - Panchakarma
13. Diet
14. Herbal food supplements
15. Rasayana
16. Behavior
17. Jyotish
18. Yagya
19. Environment
20. World health/world peace

This list is taken from the pamphlet published by Maharishi Ayurveda Medical Association of the USA, 1993.

How diets can help in balancing Doshas

Diet is one of the most important therapeutic modalities, according to Maharishi Ayurveda. Like most Ayurvedic treatment approaches, the diet is tailored according to the individual needs and is based on the assessment of the constitutional type and the imbalances that may be present in the physiology at any given time.

Maharishi Ayurveda classifies all foods into six tastes, which form the basis for a healthy diet. Inherent in each taste are certain properties that have an effect on the Doshas. Because each taste affects the Doshas differently, in order to prescribe a balanced diet all six tastes should be included in every meal, or at least once every twenty-four hours. Special Ayurvedic teas and flavorings (called *churnas*) have also been developed to assist in this process.

Classification of food: Ayurvedic perspective

All foods can be divided into six classifications based upon the six tastes of food. They are not based upon caloric value or the protein, fat, and carbohydrate content. For example:

Sweet taste: Sugar, milk, butter, rice, breads, pasta

Sour taste: Yogurt, lemon, cheese

Salty taste: Salt

Pungent taste: Spicy food, ginger, hot peppers, cumin

Bitter taste: Spinach, other green leafy vegetables, turmeric

Astringent taste: Beans, lentils, pomegranate.

Different foods have different effects on our Doshas. In the next several lines, I describe how food is prescribed based on the imbalances present at any given time.

<u>Vata imbalance</u>

One should eat more sweet, sour, and salty foods.
One should avoid pungent, bitter, and astringent foods.

<u>Pitta imbalance</u>

One should eat more sweet, bitter, and astringent foods.
One should avoid pungent, sour, and salty foods.

<u>Kapha imbalance</u>

One should eat more pungent, bitter, and astringent foods.
One should avoid sweet, sour, and salty foods.

Guidelines for improving digestion

Besides giving guidelines for diet, Maharishi Ayurveda offers recommendations for improving digestion. The power of digestion is considered very important in Ayurveda. It is as important as the food we eat. This is based upon the fact that no matter how careful you might be in the selection of food, if you cannot properly digest the food, you would not be able to assimilate and utilize the nutrients contained in it.

Following are the guidelines to improve digestion:

1. One should eat in a settled and quiet atmosphere. One should not work, read or watch TV during meals. One should always sit to eat.

2. One should eat at approximately the same times each day.

3. One should not eat too quickly or too slowly.

4. One should eat to about three-fourths of one's capacity, not leaving the table either hungry or very full.

5. One should avoid taking a meal until the previous meal has been digested. One should allow approximately three to six hours between meals and not eat unless one is hungry. For example, if it's breakfast time and one is not hungry, skip breakfast and wait until lunch time. In other words, do not eat a late breakfast. Similarly if this is lunch time and one is not hungry, skip lunch, and wait until dinner time, and so on.

6. One can sip water or juice during meals but not in excess. Milk, however, generally should not be taken with a full meal, as it is best not to mix milk with certain tastes (especially salty and sour tastes, such as yogurt, cheese, vinegar). Milk also should not be mixed with meat or fish. In general, milk should not be taken with lunch or dinner because in those two meals food is not always sweet; it is often pungent, salty and sour or bitter. Milk may be taken with toast, cereals, or sweet-tasting foods, as is the case with breakfast.

7. One should avoid yogurt, cheese, cottage cheese, and cultured buttermilk at night.

8. It is best not to heat or cook honey.

9. One should avoid ice cold beverages or foods, as they interfere with digestion.

10. One should take a few minutes to sit quietly after eating.

Constipation - Ayurveda perspective

According to Ayurveda, constipation is a serious disease. It indicates sluggishness of the bowels and weakness of the system. If you cannot move your bowels, the gases behind the stool get trapped and start to travel backwards and upwards, thereby causing reversal of the normal mechanism. As these gases start to go up and back, they may have a negative effect on your liver, spleen, stomach, heart, lungs, throat, sinuses, and even brain in this reverse order. You may have heard that a lot of people get headaches from constipation. These people are very sensitive to these gases. If this constipation process continues, the fluid contents of the bowels start to travel backwards in (a reverse order). Most physicians know that when the bowels become obstructed, people start to vomit food and even stool.

Practical points

I have given a fair amount of the practical information about Ayurveda in this chapter. Now let us see how we can apply the Ayurvedic philosophy to our daily lives.

General level

First determine which is your Dosha imbalance (Vata, Pitta or Kapha), then plan and/or change your diet according to the Dosha imbalance. It could be of great benefit in balancing the Dosha.

Physical level

1. Digestion is one of the key elements for good energy. One must pay proper attention to preserving and maintaining the digestive process and appetite. It is possible to do so by eating according to the appetite and hunger.

2. Avoid constipation: It is a serious disease and the root cause of multiple diseases. It is a challenge to avoid constipation. Taking laxatives and stool softeners can help you move your bowels, but

neither does it remove the constipation, nor does it correct the weakness or the imbalance of the system.

3. Different tastes of food: Ayurveda has classified foods according to six different tastes. It is important to understand this concept and incorporate all six classifications of foods in your daily life at least every twenty-four hours or so. Most people do not understand the importance of foods that taste spicy, pungent, bitter, astringent, sweet, and sour.

4. You should not drink cold liquids, because they slow down the digestive process. This is an important concept, because you need to keep your body warm, especially in later years of life. (At Ayurvedic conferences, usually cold or iced drinks are not served.)

5. Whenever you are taking your meals, you should focus 100 percent on your meals. You should not read, watch TV or have a conversation.

6. You should do self-body massage on a daily basis, as little as five to ten minutes a day. It is important for good circulation. Self-body massage is easy to learn; audiovisual tapes are available.

7. Regulate life like a clock to help maintain good digestion and sleep.

Mental level

Relaxation is very important. Because the hustle and bustle of daily life causes tension and high blood pressure, you must learn to unwind every day with the help of relaxation, fun activities, games, and playing. Reflection of thought on a daily basis is also essential for proper planning and improving one's life.

Spiritual level

1. You must meditate on a regular basis. Meditation is one of the best techniques to create balance at every level of the body.

2. You must treat all others with kindness and respect.

3. You must speak softly and kindly with a helping attitude.

4. You must read scriptures, e.g., Gita, Bible, Koran, on a daily basis for as few as five to ten minutes per day. The importance of these scriptures is to remind you of ethical and spiritual values, which strengthen the mind and the spirit. Only the person with a healthy and strong mind and spirit enjoys lasting happiness.

Now you can appreciate from the above that by paying attention to the little details of life, you can significantly contribute to your own health and well being at the physical, mental, and spiritual levels.

Man and nature

One of the central themes of Maharishi Ayurveda is that man and nature are very closely connected. Our body is like a finely tuned clock that runs in synchronicity with the cycles of nature. There are daily, monthly, seasonal, and annual cycles that greatly influence our physiology. In the Ayurvedic daily routine, Maharishi Ayurveda gives detailed knowledge of which activity should be undertaken at what time of the day so we can closely correlate our own individual biological rhythms with the daily rhythms of nature. Let us try to understand Maharishi Ayurveda's daily routine.

Morning

Arise early in the morning.

Evacuate bowels and bladder.

Clean teeth. Clean or scrape tongue.

Perform Ayurvedic oil massages. (Everybody should learn this and do it on daily basis.)

Shave and cut nails.

Gargle with sesame oil.

Bathe or shower.

Wear clean and comfortable attire suitable to season and activity.

Eat a light breakfast (optional).

Work or study.

Do transcendental meditation (very important for mental and spiritual health and very basic for blissful living).

Afternoon

For lunch, follow a diet balance according to your body type and the current season. Ideally take your heaviest meal at lunch, when the digestive fire is strongest.

After eating, sit quietly for a few minutes.

Work or study.

Do transcendental meditation (the very basic teaching of Maharishi Ayurveda).

Evening

For supper, follow a diet balanced according to your body type and the current season.

Take a brief walk for ten to fifteen minutes.

Engage in pleasant, relaxing activity.

Go to bed early.

Ayurvedic supplements

Take Maharishi Amrit Kalash daily.

Take Maharishi Ayurveda teas and churnas at meals to ensure that your diet is balanced according to Ayurvedic principles.

Exercises

Exercise should be done at least one-half hour before meals or one to two hours after meals. Choose the appropriate exercise according to your body type and the current season.

CHAPTER THIRTY-EIGHT

Homeopathy: Healing the Body & Mind Without Side Effects

The physician's highest and only calling
is to restore the sick to health, which is called healing.

—*Samuel Hahnemann*

A clear distinction: It is good to know from the very beginning that there is one major philosophical difference between homeopathy and many medical sciences. The difference is that, whereas the focus of most (not all) medical sciences is to get rid of the disease, the focus of homeopathy is to heal the patient.

Whenever you get sick, the first question that comes to your mind is: What do I do now? Where do I go? Whom should I call? What treatment options do I have? Can I be cured? Is cure different from palliation? These questions are natural and very genuine.

Mahatma Gandhi used to say, "Homeopathy cures more patients than any other medical science." Homeopathy is the safest or at least one of the safest medical sciences of the past 200 years in history. Homeopathy is the only medical science in which healing happens at both the physical and mental levels simultaneously.

Objectives

1. Homeopathy is the healing medical science that offers cure without the side effect of drugs.

2. Homeopathy heals not only at the physical level, but also at the mental and emotional levels.

3. Every person should read and explore what homeopathy has to offer. Almost any keen person can learn at least first aid in homeopathy to their advantage with little training.

Introduction

History: Inception of homeopathy

Homeopathy is an approximately 200-year-old medical science that was founded by Samuel Hahnemann, a German physician also known as father of homeopathy. He was a very keen observer of exceptional intelligence. The inception of homeopathy has a unique history. Dr. Hahnemann once developed every symptom of a disease known as gonorrhea without having any sexual encounter. On analyzing, it struck to him that when he goes for a morning walk, he was in the habit of chewing leaves of a certain shrub, known as *Thuja Occidentalis*. Then he realized that his condition could have been the result of chewing those leaves. This is what brought an inner awakening.

On performing further experiments, he observed that the extracts of the leaves of the plant could cure gonorrhea or discharge from the penis without having any side effects. He also observed that even if he used the diluted extract of those leaves, he continued to have similar positive results.

The dilution process is one of the essential components in preparation of homeopathic remedies, as you shall learn later in this chapter. Homeopathic remedies are prepared by the process of dilution and succussion. This process is carried to the stage that no chemical element is left in the remedies (medicine) when dispensed to the patient, therefore making these remedies safe and chemical-free. This was one of the big breakthroughs.

He further observed that homeopathic preparation of cinchona or quinine had similar effects on malaria. When quinine is given to malaria patients in conventional doses (allopathic medicines are very concentrated), patients do recover from malaria but are left with very significant side effects. One of the major side effects of quinine is that a marked residual weakness, which lasts for months and in some cases for years. Furthermore he concluded that when cinchona (the bark of quinine) is used in homeopathic preparation, it could cure malaria without leaving any residual weakness. Although he noted that quinine in homeopathic doses did not cure all cases of malaria, he needed to find different remedies for the remainder of the cases.

Then he experimented with several other medicines or remedies on similar principles. Thereafter he founded a science known as "homeopathy," which is based on "like cures like." It is important to know that homeopathic remedies, when prepared according to the homeopathic principles and used according to homeopathic guidelines, can cure multiple diseases without any side effects.

Dr. Hahnemann wrote the first book, *The Organon,* in 1810, which summarizes the principles of homeopathic science, as follows:

1. A medical cure is brought about in accordance with certain laws of healing that are natural.

2. Nobody can cure outside of these laws. (Differentiate cure from relief and palliation.)

3. There are no diseases as such, but only diseased individuals.

4. An illness is always dynamic by nature; therefore the remedy also must be dynamic in nature, if it is to cure.

5. The patient needs only one particular remedy and no other at any given stage of the illness. Unless that certain remedy is found, the patient is not cured; at best their condition is only temporarily relieved.

Homeopathic philosophy

Man does not become sick in part. When a man is sick, he is sick in the body and mind. Therefore the healing also must happen at the level of body and mind. However the disease can manifest in the physical body or in the mind.

Homeopathy: Three principles

Homeopathy has three principles or tenets. These have remained unchanged over the centuries. The truth continually re-demonstrates through successful treatment of the sick. These are as follows:

The first principle is *similia similibus curentur*, a Latin phrase meaning, "like cures like." It is known as the "law of similar."

The second principle of homeopathy is the single remedy. No matter how many symptoms a patient may be suffering from at any given time, they will need one and only one remedy. Only that remedy will cure all of their symptoms. For example, say a patient is suffering from constipation, headaches, fever, chills, and sweating; he/she will need only one remedy, not two or three to cure all the symptoms.

The third principle of homeopathy is the minimum dose. (Dilution and succussion)

Let us expand a little more on the first principle, the law of similar. The law of similar means two similar things, conditions or diseases cannot co-exist. When a homeopathic remedy is administered to a patient on homeopathic principles, it produces a condition which is very much like the disease itself. Since the condition produced by homeopathic remedies is stronger than the disease, and since two similar diseases cannot co-exist, the disease is expelled. Now we have a patient with a condition similar to the disease but produced by the remedy. We all know that the effect of the remedies is short-lived. As soon as the effect of the remedy disappears, the patient is cured of their condition. This is the law of similar.

This law is not unique or strange, even to modern medicine. Ritalin and other stimulants are used for the condition known as Attention Deficient Disorder (ADD) and or Hyperactivity Attention Deficient Disorder (HADD). I could quote many such examples.

Please note whereas homeopathy is based on law of similar, conventional medicine (allopathy) is based on "law of contraries," i.e., the opposite cures the opposite. Let us understand the law of opposites or contraries. According to this law, we need to do the opposite. For example, if the patient is dry, wet him. If he is wet, dry him. If he is cold, warm him up. If he is hot, cool him down. It has been observed that in real life the law of contraries only relieves symptoms, but does not cure the patient of the diseased condition.

Not diagnosis-oriented

Homeopathic remedies are not specific for the diagnosis or name of the disease. That means the pathological diagnosis of the disease in terms of malaria, pneumonia, diarrhea, cold, blood pressure, headaches, or heart disease has little or no therapeutic value. For example, if a physician is faced with ten cases of pneumonia or ten cases of diarrhea, each patient may get a different remedy, because the prescription will be based on the symptoms of the patient, and not on the diagnosis of the disease.

Homeopathic literature

One thing unique about homeopathic literature is that it does not change because it is all true knowledge. Truth never changes, although more and more information is added every day to the existing knowledge.

Diagnosis in homeopathy

In homeopathy much stress is put on the symptoms with which patients express their condition. Symptoms can be the physical, mental, emotional, and so on. Homeopathy believes that pathology does not express the disease of the patient in total and hence is of less importance.

There are several reasons why symptoms are so important: 1) they are the real expressions of the patient; 2) they express not only the disease, but also how the patient perceives their disease or condition, therefore symptoms have deeper meaning than the disease itself; 3) they are precursors of the pathology, hence they appear before the pathology. In other words, almost most diseases can be diagnosed and treated before pathology appears; and 4) homeopathic remedies are prescribed on a clinical diagnosis, not on a pathological diagnosis. Pathology could be of help, but is not the sole prescribing factor.

For example, a patient comes to the doctor's office and claims he is sick, yet all lab tests are negative. Now comes the test of the homeopathic physician. The homeopathic physician would not tell the patient that sickness is all in their head. The homeopathic physician knows that if the patient is in his office, they must be sick. The homeopathic doctor has to diagnose the condition before the pathology appears just by the symptoms of the patient.

Homeopathic remedies

What is unique and peculiar of homeopathic remedies (medicine)?

1. The dynamization or potentization of remedies (medicine)
2. Primary and secondary effects of the remedies (medicine)
3. Emotional and intellectual properties of the remedies
4. The amount required to prepare medicines, a comparative study

The dynamization or potentization of remedies (medicine)

Homeopathy believes that all elements in nature at physical level also have a dynamic, intellectual, and/or emotional state.

1. To bring out the dynamic and intellectual state of any physical element, it has to be prepared according to the principles of homeopathy.

2. The homeopathic art of preparation includes two simultaneous processes known as dilution plus shaking vigorously. Shaking vigorously is known as the process of succussion. The advantage of this process is that as the process is carried out further and further, it causes evolution of dynamic properties of the element, including the mental and emotional component of the remedies, which can be used for the benefit of the patient. The process of dilution makes the remedy chemical-free and hence free of causing side effects. What a breakthrough!

Primary and secondary effects of conventional medicine (not applicable to homeopathy)

In conventional medicine every drug has primary and secondary effects. For example, when we prescribe a stimulant to a patient (as in depressive), initially the medicine will have stimulating effects but when the medicine wears off, it will often exert a depressing reaction. Similarly when a sedative or tranquilizer is prescribed to the patient, as in the case of anxiety disorder or mania, initially it will have a calming effect, but when the medicine wears off, it can have a stimulating or irritating reaction. However, this is not the case of homeopathic remedies. In other words, homeopathic remedies do not have a secondary effect. This is one of the many other advantages of homeopathic remedies.

Emotional and intellectual properties of homeopathic remedies

It has been observed that when remedies are prepared on homeopathic principles from any element, e.g., minerals, plants, or animals, this causes the evolution of emotions and intellectual components of those elements from which the remedies are prepared. The plant remedies show sensitivity; the mineral remedies manifest rigidity; and the animal remedies manifest emotional and intellectual properties.

These corresponding properties of homeopathic remedies can be used for the benefit of the patient. This is also one of the unique advantages of homeopathic remedies.

The amount needed to prepare a medicine – a comparative study

The method of preparation of homeopathic medicines or remedies is quite different when compared to conventional medicine. The difference is so vast that not only the amount required to make the medicine varies a great deal, but also the side effects.

Here are examples of two medicines that are common in all the three branches of healing: conventional, Ayurvedic, and homeopathic. These are iron and quinine. Let us start with iron. In the conventional preparation of iron, a significant amount of it is required. However in the homeopathic preparation of iron, the amount required is so small that from just one iron tablet of conventional medicine, one can make homeopathic iron preparations for several thousand patients.

The amount of iron required for Ayurvedic preparation will be somewhere between the two, but much closer to the conventional doses than the homeopathic doses.

Now let's take the example of quinine or cinchona. In conventional medicine the quinine is prepared from the alkaloids in the lab. In Ayurvedic preparation, the cinchona bark of the tree is combined with other herbs to counter the side effects of the bark. To make the homeopathic quinine or cinchona preparation for thousands of patients, one does not need even one gram of cinchona bark. It is all due to the process of dilution and succussion used in preparing the homeopathic remedies.

Source of the remedies

There are more than 2,000 remedies that come from each and every source. These come from plants, minerals, animals, and other biological products. The animal kingdom includes sea animals, birds, and wild animals. Because animals have elements of emotion, anger, jealousy, and hate, animal remedies are more popular when a patient has elements of the emotions to match the symptoms of the condition of the patient.

Testing (proving) of homeopathic remedies

Homeopathic remedies, after being prepared on homeopathic principles, are proven (tested) and tried on intelligent human beings, e.g., doctors, nurses, or unpaid volunteers.

These are not experimented on animals for several reasons. The most important reason is that animals cannot express their mental and emotional aspects clearly. You see, in homeopathy the mental and emotional aspects are most important.

Testing of homeopathic remedies has only positive effects on the health of volunteers. There are no negative side effects or consequences. When homeopathic remedies are given to these volunteers, a temporary diseased state or condition is produced that soon disappears.

Now if any other patient comes along with those symptoms, which testers have experienced, then that remedy will cure that condition or disease of the patient. These probers (people) have one thing in common: They want to contribute something to the society and to the well being of the sick; therefore I would like to call them humanitarian.

Administration of homeopathic remedies (vs. allopathic)

Safety

There is not a single homeopathic remedy that is toxic; therefore these remedies can be given safely to anyone, irrespective of age, sex, or condition. These can be prescribed safely to pregnant mothers, newborn babies, or comatose patients; whereas in allopathic (conventional) medicine, there is not even a single medicine that is 100 percent safe. Almost all of these medicines have a warning that they may not be safe for pregnant woman or nursing mothers or little children.

Administration

Homeopathic remedies are easy to administer. They are administered under the tongue and are sweet to the taste. Not only are these easy to administer, but children also love them because of the taste. These remedies can be given to a vomiting patient or even comatose patients, because these remedies are absorbed through the tongue and do not need to enter the stomach.

Contraindications

There are no contraindications in homeopathy, provided the homeopathic remedies are prescribed on homeopathic principles.

Preparation of homeopathic medicines

It is very interesting to know how homeopathic remedies are prepared. The preparation of these remedies is based on dynamitization principles, which include two simultaneous processes: dilution and shaking of the remedies vigorously. Shaking vigorously is known as of process of succussion.

Basic steps in preparing homeopathic remedies

Step 1

A solution is attained from matter (plants, minerals, animals or biological products). Let us call this solution "X."

Step 2

Now one part of solution "X" is taken and diluted with 99 parts of alcohol and shaken vigorously for a certain length of time. This solution is labeled as "Remedy X Potency 1C."

Step 3

Then one part of "Remedy X Potency 1C" is diluted with 99 parts of alcohol and again shaken vigorously for a certain length of time. This solution is labeled as "Remedy X Potency 2C." (Did you notice that the potency has increased from 1C to 2C?)

Step 4

Similarly one part of "Remedy X Potency 2C" is diluted with 99 parts of alcohol and again shaken vigorously for a certain length of time. This solution is labeled as "Remedy X Potency 3C." (Now the potency has increased from 2C to 3C.)

Step 5

This process is repeated 30 times, 100 times, 1,000 times or even 100,000 times until the desired potency is attained.

When these homeopathic remedies are dispensed to the patient, the actual elements from which these remedies are prepared cannot be detected by conventional method of analysis. However remedies can be analyzed using advanced techniques, such as spectroscopic analysis.

There are several pharmaceutical companies in the United States that manufacture and dispense homeopathic remedies to physicians and pharmacies in the U.S. and across the world.

Benefits

In this world everybody wants the best, and why not? We deserve the best. To get the best, one needs to learn what is best there. What is cure? What is palliation? How do cure and palliation differ? Which medical science offers the cure without the side effects of the drugs?

First aid kit in homeopathy

If you are interested in exploring homeopathy further, you can start with using homeopathy first aid. Then you can also learn to use the bio-chemic remedies, and from thereon you can expand your horizon. Bio-chemic remedies are called tissue salt and are based on the homeopathic principle.

Buying and experimenting with a homeopathic first aid kit is safe, and it gives a little insight into homeopathic remedies. This kit may cost you from fifty to a hundred dollars. You will not become a homeopathic doctor with the first aid kit, but you will have a better understanding what all is available in the medical world.

There are approximately 2,000 homeopathic remedies that need the expertise of a physician to administer, but with the first aid kit, there are approximately 30 remedies that are commonly used. A person of average intelligence can learn to use them without any fear and often with good and positive results for common day-to-day ailments. Remember this is only a first aid kit; if you are really sick you should call a doctor.

Review of some cases and examples

I practice conventional (allopathic) medical science, homeopathy, and medical hypnosis. I find that these healing arts are complementary to each other. There is no competition among these healing medical sciences. One healing medical art can fill the gap where another healing art has left a void. One needs to be open and aware.

Whereas conventional medicine is mainly focused on the physical body, physical diseases, and what is visible to the eye or the microscope, homeopathy works even before the pathology appears. For example, a patient states "I don't feel good. I feel run down, and my all test results are negative." Here homeopathy is superb. (Please also note that the medical hypnosis is based upon the self-empowerment of the mind.)

Homeopathy is also great in emotional diseases such as fear, anxiety, jealousy, hate, anger, and diseases caused by physical or mental suppression.

Here are some cases for clarification. A twenty-three-year-old girl has been suffering from abdominal pain, constipation, and diarrhea. She was treated by a family care physician without relief. Thereafter she was referred to a gastroenterologist, and all the work-up was negative. She was diagnosed with irritable bowel syndrome but finds only symptomatic relief. She was cured by Thuja Occi and Ignatia.

A forty-seven-year-old white female came to me for the treatment of migraine headaches. She was treated by the neurologist with five HT agonist. She states that her medicine helps her headaches but she feels awful and kind of lost after taking the medicine. She was cured by Nux Vom. Her symptoms were due to business stress.

A thirty-five-year-old male comes from India with the history of weakness to the degree of exhaustion. He was treated in India with quinine for malaria. Homeopathic literature is full of similar cases where patients feel weak for months and months after an attack of malaria. He was cured with homeopathic medicine, namely china and sulfur.

All flu cases respond beautifully with oscillococcinum. It is a safe and effective flu medicine without any side effects. It is available at some health food stores. There is no such safe substitute in conventional medicine.

Night terror of children is a nightmare for the parents and frustration for the pediatrician but it is curable and manageable easily with homeopathic medicine.

Baby colic of infants is another condition that makes parents besides themselves. It is also very frustrating for the pediatrician, but is easily manageable or curable by homeopathic medicine.

Men and woman in their late fifties get joint pain and stiffness in the morning. It happens before they develop a case of arthritis. It is easily curable and manageable by homeopathic medicines.

Homeopathy is also a boon to people suffering from sub-clinical conditions and states.

These cases are just tiny examples. Homeopathy is a vast field, and you should be willing and ready to explore. Fortunately the Internet has made all of this information available with the touch of a key pad. Please look it up and make use of it.

Homeopathic associations and organizations

To find out more information about homeopathy, please contact the National Center for Homeopathic at 801 North Fairfax Street, Suite 306, Alexandria, VA 22314-1757, Phone #703-548-7790. You may also contact the American Institute of Homeopathic at the same address, Phone #888-445-9988. There are several more agencies or organizations that will provide similar information.

There are many homeopathic schools and colleges in the United States, Canada, UK, India, and all over the world. Homeopathic practice is in vogue all over the world except in the USA. In England (UK) the Royal family is one of the greatest promoters of homeopathy.

CHAPTER THIRTY-NINE

Natural Cure Part # I: Raising the Vitality

The words "natural cure" has a wider connotation, because natural cure includes many varied treatments, modalities, or methods, but things that differentiates natural cure from other methods are:

1. Its main focus is on raising the vitality of the patient.

2. The patient usually gets cured of the disease or at least makes progress in that direction.

3. Use of drugs or chemicals is strongly discouraged, although not prohibited.

In the next three chapters, I shall discuss natural healing methods extensively. From this information you should get a fairly good idea as to how natural cure differs from conventional methods. But most importantly, you will learn to use the practical information without any help, guidance or any fear and/or complications.

Objectives

1. Vitality: understanding that decrease in vitality is the primary cause of all diseases.

2. Infection, inflammation, degeneration, tumors, and stress are secondary causes of disease (and not primary).

3. In order to cure (differentiate from palliation), you must focus on the primary cause of the disease (i.e., raising the vitality) and not on the secondary causes.

Understanding natural healing methods

Introduction

All natural healing methods are based on the philosophy of raising the vitality of the patient. It does not exclude the use of medicines or drugs, if needed. It does require a disciplined way of life and full personal involvement of the patient in their care.

In natural healing methods, cure is a real possibility. However, that is not the case with most conventional methods.

The outcome of the natural cure depends on correct guidance, positive mental attitude, mental resilience, perseverance, self confidence, and introspection.

Doctors (healers) work just as guides or walk through the treatment.

Natural cure is nothing foreign to us. Nobody goes to the doctor for every little rash, headache, cold or every little cut, every little anxiety or stressful episode.

Now let us try to address the following questions:

1. What are the causes of sickness/disease?
2. What are the primary and secondary causes of disease?
3. What is healing?
4. What is the difference between healing (cure) vs. palliation?
5. What is vitality?
6. What is the role of vitality?
7. How do you raise vitality?
8. What role does our diet play in healing?

The science of natural healing is based on the fact that as long as you have good vitality, you should enjoy perfect health. However, when your vitality goes down, then and then only do the infection, inflammation, stress, and tumors start to attack you. In other words:

Good vitality means good health.

Low vitality means poor health.

Hence infection, inflammation, tumor, stress, and so on are not the primary causes but the secondary causes of disease. This is one of the chief differentiating points between the philosophy of natural healing, homeopathy, and Ayurveda vs. conventional methods of healing.

The science of natural healing believes in the concept that all the diseases originate *de novo*, i.e., they arise within the body's systems because of improper functioning of the body as a result of the decreased vitality. Ayurvedic and homeopathic arts of healing have a similar philosophy.

Take the example of a patient who has kidney stones. According to natural, homeopathic or Ayurvedic philosophy, the patient has kidney stones because their kidneys are not strong enough or their urine is not healthy enough; otherwise, there should be no reason for kidney stones.

Now let us take the example of a patient with gallstones. According to the natural art of healing, the patient has gallstones because their liver is not functioning adequately or their bile is not healthy enough; otherwise there is no reason for gallstones. In conventional medicine, the whole focus is on removing the kidney stones or the gallstones.

Similarly if a person gets cancer, tuberculosis or some other disease, according to the natural or homeopathic art of healing, it is believed that the vitality of the patient is low; therefore the germs or viruses have attacked the patient; hence treatment is focused on raising the vitality of the patient. However, in conventional medicine, every effort is focused in removing the pathology or killing the germs.

I can give several similar examples for almost every condition, but I think you can get a fairly good idea from the above information as to how different healing sciences take different approaches.

Definition

The word "cure" by definition means "to make spiritually whole." *The Oxford Dictionary* defines cure as restoration to health or to make healthy again. Natural cure also means to cure by using natural methods, with or without the use of drugs.

History of natural cure

Natural cure is an ancient art of healing. It started to evolve as early as human beings came into existence, but it became a science only at the time of Hippocrates. The first doctor really considered the father of natural cure is Dr. J. H. Tilden. He wrote a book on good healthy habits. He further writes: "We are the product of our good and bad habits/or victims of our bad habits." He also stresses that it is easy to stay healthy and prevent sickness, if you maintain good vitality.

In natural healing, many doctors have taken the use of hydrotherapy, fasting, inducing perspiration, and the use of laxatives for a very brief period of time. Other methods used in natural cure are: fruit and freshly squeezed juice diets, short vacations from the hectic life, sunbaths, liquid diets, milk diets, and so on.

How effective is natural cure?

Natural cure not only is effective, but also the cheapest, safest, and most natural way to recover from sickness or to maintain good health. It does require a disciplined way of life. The effectiveness of natural cure is directly proportional to the patient's effort, insight, and involvement in their care during the healing process. The effectiveness of natural cure can be judged by the fact, that probably it is the method of choice among philosophers, seers, and people with a good insight. These people take medicine only after the natural methods have failed.

Understanding the vital force

According to natural cure, the health of a person is a direct reflection of their vitality; the higher the vitality, the better the health, and vice versa.

The Oxford Dictionary defines vital force as the energy or spirit which animates living creatures.

Vitality is also defined as a state of being strong and active, or the power of giving continuation of life, present in all living things. Please differentiate vitality from vital signs. In the medical field, vital signs are the clinical measurements of pulse, temperature, respiration, blood pressure, and so on.

Diagnosing low vitality

A diagnosis of low vitality can be made easily by the following observations:

1. Getting sick too often
2. Having diseases that attack deeper organs of the body
3. Taking too long, to get better.
4. Having diseases that attack at an early age

<u>Getting sick too often</u>

1. When one catches cold on the slightest change of weather
2. When one gets headaches on the slightest provocation, altercation, fatigue, or stress
3. When one is prone to constipation or diarrhea on the slightest error of the diet

Diseases attack the deeper organs
When every nose cold goes to the sinuses, or when every nose cold leads to bronchitis and pneumonia, or when every urinary tract infection goes to the kidney or blood, or when every infection causes fever and chills.

Taking too long to get better
Instead of healing the wound in one week, it takes two to four weeks. Instead of getting rid of the cold in one week, it takes two to four weeks, and so on.

Having disease that attacks at an early age
It is true that we all can get sick, but it is different to have a heart attack at 40s vs. 80s, to have diabetes mellitus at the age of 30 vs. 80, to have high blood pressure at the age of 30 vs. 80, and so on.

What factors weaken our vital force or vitality?

Physical level
Built-in toxins, decreased elimination, excessive food intake, acidic food, and excessive sex, lack of sleep and rest, or excessive physical work for prolonged period of time

Mental level
Too busy a life, ignorance, lack of insight, hardships of life, mental stress and strain, no time for rest and relaxation

Spiritual level
Ego, selfishness, indifference to others not understanding life or its purpose. Anger, hate, jealousy, fear, anxiety, and worry are important causes of lowered vitality. However their importance is not properly understood by the average person.

Raising the vitality for better health: outline

Physical level

1. Eliminating toxins
2. Fasting
3. Exercising
4. Increasing rest and sleep time
5. Eliminating stress and strain
6. Alkalizing the body
7. Strengthening the digestive system

Elimination of toxins

The natural methods commonly employed in the healing process are many, but most important is the elimination of the toxins or internal waste by the four organ systems; the concept being that excessive build-up of toxins is probably one of the top causes of the decreased vitality.

Let us see how one can increase elimination of toxins by the following routes:

- Bowel movement or stool
- Urination
- Respiration
- Perspiration (skin)

Bowel movement

Constipation is considered to be one of the root causes of most acute and some chronic diseases. It is a very common problem. Constipation indicates that your digestive system is not functioning adequately. The most common causes of constipation are too much food or foods that are too acidic in nature e.g. meats, sweets, sodas, etc. Please note that for general purposes, diet soda and regular soda have similar effects in every way, except for the sugar content.

The best way to treat constipation is to provide rest to the digestive system while maintaining adequate nourishment. This is possible to do by eating fruits, juices, or cooked vegetables. These provide adequate nourishment yet are easy on the digestive system, and hence provide adequate rest to the gut. All heavy foods, such as meats and desserts, should be avoided. The use of laxatives, fiber, and stool softeners are best avoided because these neither provide strength nor rest to the digestive system.

Urination

Most people do not drink enough water, so they do not eliminate an adequate amount of urine. They are encouraged to drink more water. Tea, coffee, soda, or canned juices are best avoided. Canned juices are acidic by nature and can cause acidity and an upset stomach in some people. Only freshly squeezed juices or water is advised because these are alkaline in nature.

Excessive intake of water beyond your need can also be harmful. Do not think that drinking excessive water is always good or benign. Drinking water in excess of your need can cause weakness of the kidneys (Tao philosophy), cool the body too much in vata constitution (Ayurveda philosophy), and cause unnecessary dilution of the blood and fluid compartments of the body (conventional medicine).

Respiration

Most people do not breathe properly. They breathe shallow and fast. They are not using even 50 percent of the capacity of their lungs. One must breathe deeply and slowly in order to use the lungs to their fullest extent (See Chapter 10). Breathing deeply and slowly not only helps us get rid of more carbon dioxide, but it also stimulates the parasympathetic nervous system (and hence relaxes the mind). When we breathe deeply, we also use fewer breaths and that prolongs life; the reason being the numbers of breaths are limited for each person for their life span. (See

Chapter 10) Deep breathing also increases energy and memory and improves our digestion.

Skin
Sweating or perspiration is another source of elimination of the toxins. Your skin constitutes a fairly large area of your body. During perspiration a significant amount of toxins can be eliminated, thereby easing the burden of your lungs and kidneys.

Fasting
This is a natural way of putting the body's digestive system and mind to rest. During any sickness, the digestive system is the first to suffer. Whether malfunctioning of the digestive system is the cause or the effect of the disease may be debatable. The fact remains that the digestive system suffers and needs some kind of relief from food during sickness. Fasting provides an opportunity for the digestive system to recuperate. (See Chapter 42)

Exercise
Exercise is of the modality or method of increasing your body's heat and/or its vitality. Start with a gentle and mild exercise program and build up gradually. (See Chapter 24)

Increase rest time
Increase in sleep and rest time also increases your vitality. This fact needs due and proper and due consideration. However, because of today's busy schedule, it is becoming harder and harder to get adequate rest and sleep. Eliminate stress and strain by taking mini vacations or practicing relaxation techniques.

Strengthening your digestive system

Fruits or fruit juices (only freshly squeezed juices) are given for just two to three days. This provides nourishment to your body, and your digestive system gets relief from the hard work of digesting food. This is based on the philosophy that digestion of food is a hard process, involving several enzyme systems. Whereas digestion of the juices and fruits is an easy process and provides adequate nourishment while the digestive system has a chance to recuperate.

Raising vitality at the mental and spiritual levels

People do a hundred and one things to get better at the physical level, but do very little to strengthen or heal at the mental and spiritual levels. Healing at the mental and spiritual levels is at least as important, if not more, as healing at the physical level.

Mental level

Here one practices the art of staying calm in all circumstances and situations. The practice of observance of silence helps a great deal in achieving this goal. (See Chapter 27) Relaxation can be an extra bonus in healing.

Spiritual level

This involves getting rid of ego, observing silence, meditating; reading religious scriptures, understanding life and its purpose, caring for or bonding with others, bonding with higher self, connecting with the supreme and loving the humanity help to heal at the spiritual level. It is important to instill positive emotions, e.g., love, sincerity, truthfulness, altruism, caring, and sharing. Getting rid of negative emotions, anger, jealousy, hatred, anxieties, fears, and worries is extremely important for mental and spiritual health, and for raising vitality at mental and spiritual levels.

Practical points

Natural cure is a way of raising your vitality at the physical, mental, and spiritual levels. It requires self-involvement and a disciplined way of life. Natural healing does provide cure compared to relief obtained by most conventional methods. During natural healing, although use of conventional medicine or drugs is discouraged, they are not excluded if they become necessary. This should also make you think why not to use natural methods at least as a complement, if not a substitute, even if you choose conventional methods of healing?

The key message

Health is a direct reflection of the vitality of the individual. Good health means good vitality, and poor health means poor vitality.

Mantra

I shall keep up my vitality with a healthy diet and a balanced and calmed mind.

CHAPTER FORTY

Natural Cure Part # II Alkalize with Diet

In the previous chapter while discussing how to raise vitality, I have mentioned the importance of keeping the body alkaline. In this chapter I shall discuss what food can make the body alkaline and in what proportions these foods should be ingested.

You all know that diets play a major role in keeping us healthy. Diets are important not only for prevention of diseases and maintenance of good health, but also for curing diseases. Ayurveda, nutrition, and natural healing sciences focus a great deal on diets.

It is important to understand that all or most diseases arise in an acidic body. Conversely you should also know that an alkaline body is a healthy body and free of most diseases.

No doubt you have heard before: "We are what we eat and what we think." This aphorism has stood the test of time. As your body is the direct product of the food you eat, similarly your mind is the direct product of what you think. Interestingly your mouth is the common organ for both, i.e., you eat by mouth and also speak by mouth. Therefore you should be careful, cautious, and selective before opening the mouth, either for eating or for speaking.

Objectives

1. To understand that food is your best medicine. Diet plays a major role in the maintenance of health, prevention, and/or cure of diseases.

2. In order to keep your body healthy or alkaline, you need to eat a balanced diet and also in moderation. You should eat according to your appetite and needs, and not according to the modern formulas based on caloric needs.

Introduction

Diet has been discussed by several authors, and there is an abundance of literature on this subject, and why not? Diet has a major impact on our health and well being. To give you an idea, please note the following:

1. Your body is a direct product of the food you eat.

2. Diet can be used to gain weight (for people who are underweight and malnourished) and to lose weight (for people who are overweight).

3. Diet can be used to get rid of toxins.

4. Diet can be used for treating many diseases, acute and chronic (Ayurvedic and nutrition principles).

5. With proper selection of food you can keep the body alkaline, therefore prevent and even cure diseases.

Relationship of disease to acidity

Acidity may not be a disease in itself, but it provides the soil or medium for growth of disease. All the diseases, whether it is an inflammation, infection, degenerative or even growth, flourish in an acidic body. In other words, diseases cannot attack a healthy or alkaline body that easily. For comparison, you cannot grow a seed on a dinner plate. You have to go to the yard, put it in soil, and then water it. In other words you cannot grow seeds without water, soil, and sun. You should also know that the bacteriologist can grow bacteria only on a special medium, not on a plain dish.

Similarly mental diseases flourish only in an acidic mind. What makes the mind acidic? Negative and harmful thoughts towards self and others, e.g., anger, greed, jealously, hatred, selfishness and so on.

Keeping the body alkaline: Playing it right

Keeping the body alkaline is probably one of the top secrets of good health. It goes without saying that keeping the body alkaline raises your vitality. I have read several books in this reference, however I find that the following two books are easy to read and follow:

- *Natural Cure of Common Diseases* by Dr. Vithaldas Modi (most practical and useful information)
- *Alkalize or Die* by Dr. Theodore Abroody

The subject of keeping the body alkaline will be discussed in three sub-headings:

1. Eating the right quality of food.
2. Eating the right quantity of food
3. Keeping the digestive system healthy

Eating the right quality (nature) of food

Humans are supposed to eat 80 percent alkaline food and 20 percent acidic food for proper maintenance of alkalinity. Vegetables and fruits are the most natural alkaline foods on Earth.

Dr. Vithaldas Modi in his book, *Natural Cure of Common Diseases*, has tried to cure each and every disease by a vegetable and fruit diet. He has cured gonorrhea, syphilis, high blood pressure, asthma, all skin diseases, arthritis, and even infections, just by diet alone. It is worth reading his book. All the information is practical and easy to follow for an average individual. The message is very clear that whenever our body becomes acidic, we become sick. So the best way to get rid off sickness and diseases is by making the body alkaline.

Foods: acid and alkaline

Before we go further on this subject, let us understand the acidic and alkaline nature of foods. I have classified these into three categories.

1. Extremely acidic foods: either avoid or take in minimum amounts:
   Meat and poultry
   Sweets and desserts
   Alcohol (extremely acid)
   Smoking, soda, coffee, and
   Most conventional drugs/medicines

2. Mildly acidic foods: remember these foods are needed because we do need some acidic food.
   Grains and beans (eat in the amounts mentioned below)

3. Alkaline foods:
   Most fruits and vegetables

The role of fruits and vegetables in keeping the body alkaline

Fruits and vegetables are the best foods that can make the body alkaline. Fruits and vegetables are two different types of foods that you must learn to differentiate. These differ in several ways, e.g., nutritional value, digestibility, and their nature. Fruits are easier to digest and are cleansing agents but are limited in protein value. Vegetables are slightly harder to digest when compared to fruits, but have significant protein value and thus are building blocks.

On the average, your diet should consist of at least 25 to 30 percent green vegetables. Vegetables can be combined with any other type of food, whereas fruits are preferably eaten alone for best benefits. However both fruits and vegetables have mild anti-inflammatory properties because of the bioflavonoid contents in them. In other words, they act like mild aspirin or ibuprofen. This fact has very useful implications from a health point of view.

Eat the right quantity of food to keep the body alkaline

Although it is important that we eat an alkaline diet, it is equally important, if not more so, that we eat in moderation. No matter how alkaline and healthy foods may be, if taken in excess of your needs, they can also cause acidity.

Eating in moderation keeps the body healthy, even if you make slight dietetic mistakes. According to Ayurveda, eating in excess can cause the production of AMA, which is believed to be the Number One cause of most Kapha diseases. (AMA is not pronounced as A.M.A., but as one word.)

You know the phrase: "We dig our graves with our teeth." In other words, *eating in moderation should be the basic rule.*

Keeping the digestive system healthy

Good digestion and a good appetite keep the body alkaline, whereas an upset stomach or overburdened stomach can cause acidity. Therefore maintenance of good digestion in itself is an important factor in keeping the body alkaline. In this reference, please note the following:

1. Dr. Henry Beiler, M.D. in his book, *Food is Your Best Medicine*, strongly recommends that for all health purposes the heaviest meal should be lunch or breakfast and not dinner. This helps in the preservation of the appetite.

2. Eat in moderation (the key).

3. Eat only if hungry. One should never ever eat without an appetite. Eating without an appetite can also cause acidity.

4. Learn to match the degree of appetite with the amount and quality of the food eaten at any given meal. (See Chapter 9)

5. Keep the digestive system healthy. Do whatever you have to do to preserve the appetite. (Chapter 9)

6. Keep the bowels open but without the help of laxatives, stool softeners or fiber supplements.

The role of diet in health and disease

This will be discussed in two subheadings:

1. Diet in acute diseases
2. Diet in chronic diseases and for maintenance of health

Diet in acute diseases

1. Eat lightly. For example, have soup and toast, or soup and rice, or juices. Avoid animal proteins, e.g., meat, milk, and eggs, as these are hard to digest.

2. Avoid all raw foods, including salads and fruits (a little hard to digest), during acute diseases, however, you should eat these foods when you are enjoying good health.

3. Avoid acidic foods (soda, meat, desserts, pickles, and all alcoholic beverages).

4. Keep the body warm. (Eat only warm foods and cooked foods. Avoid all cold drinks.)

Diet in chronic diseases and for maintenance of good health

The role of a balanced diet is much more important in combating chronic diseases than acute diseases, because in acute diseases it is simply a matter of days and thus not a major issue. But in chronic diseases, the long-term maintenance of adequate nourishment is of special concern.

How to balance the diet

Now I shall discuss what proportion of different types of food should be eaten to create balance.

Grains

The most important ingredient of your diet should be grains. Grains can amount to 40 to 60 percent of your diet (Macrobiotic principle). Please note that grains are mildly acidic. However we do need to eat 20 percent acidic foods. The sicker you are the less acidic food you should eat. You must know that beans and grains can cause constipation, and therefore these should be eaten with vegetables.

Beans

Beans are very rich in protein and should constitute only 5 to 10 percent of your diet.

Fresh green vegetables

Fresh green vegetables should constitute 20 to 30 percent of your diet. Even when you are healthy, you should eat no less then 25 percent vegetables. If you are suffering chronically from asthma, high blood pressure, diabetes, and/or skin conditions, the importance of fresh vegetables becomes even greater and the amount eaten should be increased.

Please differentiate fruits from vegetables; these are quite different in nature. Also note that grains are not vegetables. Some people consider corn a vegetable, which is not the case. The American Cancer Society recommends five servings of fruits and vegetables daily.

Vegetables are building blocks and have some protein value, whereas fruits are cleansing and have very little protein value, so you must eat more vegetables and less fruits especially if you wish to gain weight. From the five servings of fruits and vegetables, you can have three or four servings of vegetables and one or two servings of fruits; the importance of vegetables cannot be overemphasized.

You must eat salad at least once or twice a day with lunch and/or dinner. You can imagine the nourishing value of vegetables from the simple fact that most herbivorous animals, e.g., rabbits, cows, horses, elephants, giraffes, and others depend on grass and leaves (or vegetables) to satisfy their protein, potassium, calcium, fiber, and vitamin requirements. Please note that vegetables also have mild anti-inflammatory properties because of the bioflavonoid contents in them.

Fruits

Fruits are different from vegetables. Fruits are a meal in themselves. Fruits preferably should be eaten alone, whereas vegetables can be eaten with beans, meat, or anything. Fruits have a fair amount of carbohydrates which are complex and healthy, but the carbohydrate content of vegetables is generally low. Keep in mind that fruit juices are quite rich in sugar.

Animal proteins

Animal proteins include but aren't limited to meat, fish, chicken, and eggs. Milk is also an animal protein but is alkaline in nature. Because animal proteins are very acidic in nature, they should be eaten in small quantities and preferably with vegetables and not with grain or beans. For example, do not eat a cheeseburger or chicken sandwich or cold sandwiches, but you can eat just the burger with vegetables, or the chicken with vegetables or fish with vegetables.

Meat causes some sort of irritation or mild inflammation in the system of many individuals. Furthermore, meat is poor in magnesium, potassium, calcium, minerals, and fibers. Meat is also rich in salt, cholesterol, and fat, and can cause constipation.

Ayurvedic system of healing: Foods by taste

In the Ayurvedic system of healing, foods are not prescribed based on grains, beans, vegetables, or meat. Nor is it based on protein, carbohydrates, and fat values, but rather on the taste of the food.

All foods are classified into six types. These are: sweet, sour, salty, bitter, pungent, and astringent. When you eat in excess any class of food, it causes imbalance in the system. In the U.S., people eat an excess of sweet-tasting foods and ignore the importance of bitter, pungent, sour, and spicy foods. So choosing foods of all different tastes for your daily diet is essential for proper balance.

In Ayurveda, every patient is prescribed a diet whenever they visit the doctor, based on the imbalances at that given time. (See Chapter 40)

- In Vata imbalance, more salty, sour, and sweet-tasting foods are recommended.
- In Pitta imbalance, more bitter, astringent, and sweet foods are recommended.
- In Kapha imbalance, one is advised to eat more pungent, astringent, and bitter foods. Most of the diseases which are structural in nature have Kapha imbalance.

<u>Water</u>

You should drink an adequate amount of water. Not drinking an adequate amount of water, or drinking too much water, can be harmful. According to the philosophy of Taoism, drinking an excessive amount of water can cause weakness in the kidneys. It is also interesting to note that in the treatment of high blood pressure, diuretics or (water pills) are first line of drugs. According to the Ayurvedic principle of healing, excessive water can have a negative effect on individuals with a Vata constitution.

Do not mix more than one protein at a time.

1. A cheeseburger is not kosher or healthy, because it mixes two proteins. You can verify this with any Jewish friend. Either eat a cheese sandwich or eat a burger, not both at the same time.

2. Don't eat hamburger with milk. Again these are two different types of protein in one meal.

3. Don't eat fish with milk.

4. Don't eat a cheese omelet. Eat either cheese or an omelet. Don't mix the two.

5. Don't eat eggs with bacon.

Do not mix proteins with carbohydrates.

Don't eat meat with gravy, carbohydrates, and/or bread. You should avoid all meat sandwiches. When you eat meat, it is preferable to eat it with vegetables, not with fruit or carbohydrates, such as potatoes or bread. You should eat a burger without the bread or a hot dog without the bread. To quote a familiar marketing slogan, "Think outside the bun." That is, don't eat the bun with the burger or the hot dog!

Case studies

Here are some examples of patients. You can appreciate how each patient was cured by a simple change in diet. Please also know that no other change was made in the treatment regime.

Patient # 1

Prickly heat: Patient states he is a vegetarian. Patient complains of rashes, itching, burning and even urticaria. Now let us analyze the diet of the patient:

Breakfast – Milk and cereal (milk or bread) or bread and pickles with tea (acidic)

Lunch – Bread, beans and yogurt, dessert (acidic combination)

Dinner – Bread, beans, some vegetables (not always), yogurt

Bedtime – Milk

Analysis: Although a vegetarian, his diet is extremely acidic.

Diet prescription: 60 percent vegetables cooked or raw, 15 percent fruits, 20 percent grains and 5 percent beans.

Results: In two weeks a 100 percent cure.

Patient # 2

Malaria: Patient is a twenty-five-year-old male. Patient has been treated with quinine. Now he suffers from weaknesses as a result of both. Let us analyze his diet:

Breakfast – Cheese omelet and bread

Lunch – Fish or chicken sandwich

Dinner – Red meat, potatoes, tea, dessert, occasionally vegetables

Bedtime snack – Cookies

Analysis: Extremely acidic diet lacking in vegetables and fruits

Diet prescription: 60 percent vegetables, 20 percent fruits, 5 percent beans, and 15 percent grains

Result: Cure in four weeks, no weakness, no disease

Patient # 3

Diabetes: Patient is a fifty-year-old male, 350 pounds, newly diagnosed, presented with the infection of the scrotum with tendency to gangrene.

Patient was admitted to the hospital and blood sugar brought under control with insulin. Later on he was given an alkaline diet and was advised to lose weight. He was informed that he could be cured of diabetes if he loses weight and eats plenty of vegetables.

Analysis: Patient diet was extremely acidic. His diet was rich in meat and carbohydrates and poor in vegetables and fruits.

Diet prescription: 60 percent vegetables, 20 percent fruits, 15 percent grains, and 5 percent beans

In 3 months, patient lost 50 pounds and had no more diabetes.

Type II diabetes usually can be cured in many cases, if patient loses weight and follows an alkaline diet.

Patient # 4

Burning and frequency of urination: Patient is a thirty-year-old male; the problem has persisted for four weeks.

Diet

Breakfast – Cereal with little milk, coffee and orange juice

Lunch – Fish sandwich and Coke

Dinner – Beer, meat, bread, and tomatoes

Analysis: very acidic diet

Diet advice: 60 percent vegetables, 20 percent fruits, 20 percent grains

Result: cured in two weeks

Patient # 5

Eczema: History of rash all over the body that itches intensely in the evening after eating a heavy dinner

Diet

Breakfast – Tea and toast

Lunch – Fish or cheese sandwich

Dinner – Meat and potatoes followed by dessert and coffee

Analysis: extremely acidic diet

Prescription: 60 percent vegetables, 20 percent fruit, 15 percent grains, 5 percent beans

Result: Patient cured in two weeks.

Some important observations

These case studies teach us one thing that: how easy it is to fall sick by the excessive intake of acidic foods. It is also important to understand that a vegetarian diet also can be acidic, if not properly planned. You must differentiate a vegetarian diet from vegetables.

A vegetarian diet does not mean the diet is balanced, as you have seen in above examples. A vegetarian also suffers from diseases because they have the wrong concept about the diet. When I say vegetables, I mean fresh, green, leafy vegetables (lettuce, spinach, asparagus, broccoli, dandelion and collard greens, carrots). Eggplant has a different effect and should not be eaten in excess, whereas green leafy vegetables can be eaten in abundance.

According to macrobiotics, chewing plays an important role in the digestion of food. It makes lot of sense because saliva is alkaline in nature, which is especially important for the digestion of the carbohydrates. In order to keep the body alkaline, not only do you have to eat an alkaline diet, but also you need to eat in moderation, at the right time (when hungry), and chew your food well.

Benefits

Remember all or most diseases arise in an acidic body. It is hard for diseases to survive in an alkaline body. Whenever you are victim of any ailments, focus on making the body more alkaline. The following guidelines will help you to regain good health or make the body more alkaline.

- Avoid all acidic foods:

A. All animal protein (fish, chicken, egg, meat)
B. All alcoholic beverages
C. Coffee and tea
D. All carbonated beverages

E. All sweets, desserts, and pickles

- Fast and/or eat lightly for few days (See Chapter 44). Because vegetables and fruit are alkaline, their intake should be increased. In acute diseases, you may not eat raw vegetables or fruits, because they are hard to digest. However you can have vegetable soups and light food.
- In chronic diseases, your intake of raw vegetables and fruits should be increased. Examples of chronic diseases are asthma, skin diseases, diabetes, and heart disease. If you have a problem digesting vegetables, you may slightly cook or steam them.
- You may eat brown rice for several days, in addition to vegetables, if you have a big appetite.
- You must chew your food well. (Chewing increases the alkalinity of the body because saliva is alkaline in nature.)

The key message

In order to keep the body healthy, you need to keep it alkaline. Vegetables and fruits are foods that can make the body alkaline. Eating in moderation when combined with an exercise program can also help keep the body alkaline or healthy. One can also keep the body and mind alkaline by thinking good, beneficial, and positive thoughts.

Mantra

An alkaline body is a healthy body, and I will keep mine alkaline. Eating in moderation and/or eating the alkaline foods (fruits and vegetables) can keep my body alkaline. Also an alkaline mind is a healthy mind. Positive and beneficial thoughts are the best way to keep the mind alkaline.

CHAPTER FORTY-ONE

Healing (Self-healing)

Healing means becoming whole or complete. It can happen only when you are fully involved in your care with faith, determination, and commitment. No medicine, doctor, or hospital can heal or cure you without your full commitment. Please also differentiate healing (cure) from palliation (relief).

How many times have you heard about people that were diagnosed with cancer and were told that they had only three to six months to live? The patients left the hospital out of disappointment and frustration, took charge of their health, came back after six months or a year later, and surprised everyone, including their physician. It does not happen often, but it does happen.

I am not suggesting that if you have cancer, you should leave the hospital and start healing on your own. But I am suggesting that you should always be 100 percent involved in your care to get the best results. You should listen to every word of advice and do everything possible wholeheartedly and without reservation, and with full faith, determination, and commitment. Your body does have healing power. Magic can and does happen!

Healing is akin to all living beings. All living beings are different from non-living things by their ability to eat, grow, reproduce, think, and most importantly to heal. Probably healing is one of the most important qualities of living beings. Every living entity, whether it is a cell, bacteria, virus or any life from the smallest being to the biggest creature, has built-in intelligence to heal; the higher the degree of the intelligence the better the ability to heal. Since human beings are the most intelligent creatures on Earth, you can imagine the healing power that they must possess.

Objectives

1. To understand what healing is, and how it differs from palliation or relief

2. Every intelligent and conscious being have the power to heal him/herself.

3. One needs to get involved 100 percent in their care with body, mind, and spirit in order to get healed or to get the best results.

Definition

According to the dictionary, healing (cure) means "to make spiritually whole or complete." Healing can also be defined as the returning of the body's functions to normal as before the diseased state. Remember healing or cure is very different from palliation or relief of symptoms.

If you have to take medicine on an ongoing basis, that is not cure. You can call it only palliation. Examples are people who take medicine on daily basis for diabetes, arthritis, high blood pressure, asthma, cholesterol problems, migraine headaches, and so on.

Introduction

You must have observed that some people rarely get sick, and if they do, they bounce right back as if they know how to heal. Spiritual people not only heal themselves but also heal others. Healing is akin for all living beings.

Degree of healing

Healing means becoming complete or whole. Only very few people achieve that goal. One of the reasons is that healing at least in part is based upon expectation. For the sake of understanding, if we can grade healing from one to five, some people will be satisfied at level two, whereas most people will be satisfied at level three or four. People who have faith in themselves will continue to work towards healing until they achieve 100 percent of their goal.

Why some people don't heal or get better

It is interesting and intriguing that although everybody wants to be healed or cured only very few people really succeed in the mission. There are several reasons for that:

Ignorance

This is probably one of the top causes. Ignorance can be at several levels. Most people do not understand what is meant by healing. There are very few people who would be able to differentiate between palliation and cure. Most people would also have a hard time explaining whether they are healthy or sick.

Secondly, most people seek easy solutions. They go to the health spa, health store, or nutrition stores looking for vitamins, organic foods, or supplements to get healthy. Health and happiness do not come in bottles or in vitamins, minerals, supplements or even in health spas. Those people who are looking for solutions in the health food store are not addressing even one-third of the problem; in reality they are at a loss. I want to tell them that the good health pill has not yet been invented as yet, nor is it expected to arrive soon.

Furthermore most people are focused only on the body. There are very few people who understand the concept of body, mind, and soul.

Mental and spiritual health is really the basic foundation of health and happiness, although it is true that physical health is essential and an integral part of total health. So in order to enjoy perfect health, you have to be healthy at all three levels. Even if one of the elements is missing, you will not be able to heal completely.

For better understanding, let me give you an example of cake making. Let us check the ingredients we need to make a cake: Flour, water, eggs, sugar, butter, oven, and the recipe. If any of the ingredients is missing, you will not be able to make the cake.

Likewise if you want to heal, you have to incorporate each and every ingredient into the health program, i.e., physical, mental, and spiritual. In other words, just taking care of your body without paying any attention to the mind and soul is not going to make you healthy or happy.

Laziness and procrastination

Probably this is the next important reason why some people do not heal. They keep on postponing until it is too late.

Fate (luck): Misbelief

Some people do very little for themselves, and they don't even seek medical help, while others refuse to take medicine. They leave everything to fate or luck.

Mercy of others

Some people, due to ignorance, leave everything at the mercy of God, the doctors, or others.

All the above factors point out only one thing: that ignorance or lack of self-involvement is the most important reason for not healing.

Basic tenets of true healing

1. Understanding the healing power of the body and mind
2. Need awareness for body and its functions
3. Faith
4. Self-involvement
5. Effort and outcome
6. Self-healing vs. healing others

Understanding the healing power of the body

According to Ayurveda, our body is autonomous, i.e., self-governing, self-diagnosing, and self-regulating. That means it is capable of diagnosing and healing on its own. It is due to the inherited intelligence in the body.

Observe the instinct of animals. Even animals have some degree of awareness. When carnivorous animals get sick or diseased, they suspend their regular meat diet and resort to chewing certain plants or grass for a brief a period to induce vomiting or to give rest to their stomach in order to heal.

Furthermore in almost all acute diseases, everybody gets better. It may take a little shorter or longer, depending on the vitality of the person. The more one gets involved in their care, the faster they get better. Nobody can afford to run to the doctors for every little rash, cold and ache. If you get a paper cut or little wound, you don't run to the doctor. You make sure that you have been immunized against tetanus. You cover the wound, and it heals in the due course of time. (Covering the wound is important for healing so that no bugs or viruses can get in.)

Don't take pride in showing your wound to your friends and relatives, because they will look at the wound and say, "Oh, my God" or "Wah!" Thus they bless you with the germs of their mouth. (The human mouth is the reservoir of the worst germs.)

Let us take some more examples. You get bitten by a mosquito or by your dog. Usually all that is required is for you to cleanse the wound and cover it up.

If you get diarrhea, you should stick to the B.A.R.T. diet (Bananas, Applesauce, Rice or Toast), take fluids to prevent dehydration, and you will be okay.

Similarly, if you have a mild cough, just fast for a day or two, and follow the diet that I have prescribed in this book and you will be okay. (But if you get a cough and continue to eat three full meals a day despite your body's plea in the form of loss of appetite, your disease will be protracted. You may need a chest x-ray, antibiotics, cough medicine, sleeping medicine, and so on.)

Awareness of the body and its functions

The more conscious and aware you are of your body and its functions the more easily you can heal. It is interesting to note that during good health we are not aware of our body or its functions. As in any normal or good functioning organization, nobody is aware of the good functioning of the organization. People are aware only when some malfunction happens or some problem arises. We are not aware of the head, unless we have a headache. We are not aware of our joints, unless we have joint pain. We are not aware of our lungs, unless we have difficult breathing, and so on.

Equally important and interesting is the fact that whenever we begin to pay attention to the diseased part with positive intention, that part begins to heal, as if paying attention brings energy to the part for the purpose of healing. This is a very important point to keep in mind.

Faith

Faith is important in healing. Jesus was a great healer, but he did not take every case that came to him for healing. When people came for healing, he used to ask them, "Do you really think that you can be healed?" If the people answered in the affirmative, then he used to ask them another question, "Do you think I can heal you?" If the person who wanted to be healed did not answer in the affirmative to both questions, he did not do the healing for that person. In other words, for healing to happen, one has to have full faith in oneself and in the healer.

Self-involvement

This is one of the most important elements. I often meet people who have not seen a doctor in forty or fifty years. I ask them how they take care of themselves, and they tell me they just listen to their body, and it knows what to do. Look at animals or the people in underdeveloped countries. How many internists do they have? How many obstetricians, gynecologists, and surgeons do they have? How many cancer doctors do they have? You all know that all the medical inventions and therapeutics came only in the last sixty to seventy years.

You also know that prevention and early intervention is possible only with self-involvement, so one does not wait until it is too late or until disease is too advanced

Effort and outcome

We all know that there is some degree of correlation between the two. For example if I want to get an A, I have to work harder and smarter than if I want to be content with a C, and so on. This is true everywhere in life. I can tell you from my own observation that there are only very few people who make sincere efforts in the process of healing.

Self-healing vs. healing others

Self-healing and healing others are very different from each other. Self-healing is not difficult. People of average intellect can heal as long as they listen to the needs of their body and have faith in themselves. They must also have will and determination to make changes in their lifestyle as required.

Healing others is a difficult job. It requires advanced education and training, and one must be spiritual. One must have love and compassion for others, as well.

I will give one analogy. In order to perceive God, you do not need to know Vedas, the Bible, or any scriptures. If your heart is pious or pure, have faith in yourself and persevere, you will perceive God. But if you want to teach others how to perceive God, then you may have to study Vedas, the Bible, or other scriptures.

Prevention of diseases: physical, mental, and spiritual

"An ounce of prevention is equal to a pound of cure." This is a valuable aphorism. Prevention is possible only when diseases are detected at the early onset, and you are in the habit of listening to the needs of your body.

Physical level

The digestive system usually suffers in most physical ailments. Cause and effect is not the issue here. Therefore, whenever you lose your appetite or are not digesting food properly, you should be concerned. You should get extra physical rest, and you should also rest your stomach by fasting and/or observing a light diet (soup and toast).

Mental and spiritual levels

You should also be aware of the early warning signs of mental and spiritual disease. These are restlessness, anger, greed, jealousy, fear, anxiety, worries, use of insulting and harsh language, quarreling, and intolerance. But the single most important early sign of mental and spiritual disease is the lack of happiness and inability to enjoy life.

This is a call to take action. It is the time to meet some spiritual leaders, read the Holy Scriptures, and take time for insight. You need to reflect on your life, meditate, and meet good-intentioned and wise people. You should be aware that mental and spiritual diseases or derangements can cause physical diseases and vice versa. A good upbringing during childhood, balance in life, and faith in yourself can make your mind and spirit strong and thus help in the prevention of the mental and spiritual diseases.

Treatment of diseases

The treatment of the diseases falls under two categories:

1. Physical diseases: acute and chronic
2. Mental and spiritual diseases

Physical diseases (acute and chronic)

Treatment of acute diseases

Acute diseases are those diseases that are self-limiting by nature. In acute diseases, most people do get better with little or no help. These diseases are short-lived and do not continue for a long period of time. Examples are simple colds, flu, simple fevers, body aches, diarrhea, and acute fatigue.

Whenever you have an acute disease, two things invariably happen: 1) you feel tired, and 2) you lose your appetite. This is the most important accompaniment of most acute diseases. This is the time to listen to your body's needs. You must provide more rest to your body and also to your digestive system in the form of light diet or fasting. You may have to do that for few days or as long as the illness lasts.

On the other hand, if you continue to eat regular meals and do your regular amount of work, you will not be giving your body and stomach a chance to do the reparative work. In that case, the acute disease can become chronic, protracted, or even complicated.

In summary, the treatment of acute diseases is simple. Give rest to the mind, body, and stomach. Eat simple and easily digestible food. Eat as little as you possibly can live on until the appetite returns.

Now let us look at some common examples. If you have diarrhea, follow the BART diet: Banana, Applesauce (not apples), Rice or Toast. It is important to remember that apples have a very different effect than applesauce. While the apple diet opens the bowels, applesauce has a binding effect; it is constipating. It is just the opposite of the apple diet. Also do not eat vegetables, fruits, and meat. Milk and milk products should also be avoided during diarrhea (also during a cough). Also avoid tea, coffee, colas, or drinks that have caffeine in them. You usually will be okay in twenty-four to forty-eight hours.

Now let us look at an example of an acute bronchitis. You should just stop eating regular meals, including animal proteins. You may have soup, toast, onion soup or garlic soup. You also must avoid milk and dairy products. You also must avoid bananas and cooling foods. Bananas are not a good food during bronchitis, but they are okay to eat during diarrhea. Bananas are very cooling by nature, and as such, they aggravate a cough. Also avoid cold drinks, including cold water and cold juices. Cold foods are best avoided not only in acute and chronic diseases, but in general for prevention of the diseases and maintenance of good health. This is one of the principles of Ayurveda. You should seek the help of a physician, if you are not responding to these simple measures.

Treatment of chronic diseases

Swami Parmahansa Yoganada states: "All chronic diseases have some degree of mental derangement." It is important to understand that the mind and body are directly and proportionately related to each other. In chronic disease, the problem is much more complex. Chronic diseases tend to linger. The examples of these are high blood pressure, arthritis, asthma, diabetes, heart disease, cancer, and so on.

You should know that chronic diseases do not come from the outer world. These are the results of mismanagement, suppression, or neglect of acute diseases. These chronic diseases may have some hereditary and genetic factors, too. However you should not focus or worry on that aspect as much, because these are not modifiable factors. You should also be aware that there are always some elements of mental derangement in most chronic diseases in the form of anxiety, stress, sadness, and restlessness.

Chronic diseases: How to facilitate the healing process

1. Eat light, balanced, and nourishing foods. Eat half to two-thirds of your capacity. Do not depend on soup and toast as you did in acute diseases, because in chronic diseases it is a long-term affair, and you need to get proper nourishment.

2. Do not overexert at work or at home. Working too hard at the cost of your health will slow down the healing process.

3. Get adequate physical and mental rest.

4. Maintain a gentle exercise program. An exercise program is important to maintain your vitality. However, you do not need to do heavy exercises.

5. You should have faith in yourself without which healing is difficult. Without faith, even the healer cannot heal anyone. (I often notice that people just before death lose faith and hope.)

6. Get professional help or if you are in the medical field, read medical literature in the diseases affected.

7. Keep up with your spiritual connections.

Treatment of mental and spiritual diseases

Treatment of mental and spiritual diseases is at least as important if not more as the physical diseases. Mental and physical diseases are very much interlinked with each other.

Swami Parmahnsa Yogananda has written a beautiful pocket monograph, "Scientific Healing Affirmation," that emphasizes:

A. The healing power of the mind
B. The importance of the repetition of the healing affirmation
C. The use of imagination in the healing process

Healing at the subconscious level

That is to think that my body is getting healthier or normal. Staying focused on this affirmation does help the healing process. You should never think or imagine for the disease to go away. This has a negative effect. The word disease should not come to your mind if you want to be healed. For example, we never say "I don't want to fail." Instead, we say "I want to succeed," because the words fail has a negative connotation.

Study the biographies of great people

This gives good insight. It is amazing what kind of life they have led. How much they have suffered. How they came out as a winner each time. It gives us energy, strength, and faith.

Meet spiritual people and well wishers

Read and refresh, the moral, ethical, and spiritual values that provide mental, and spiritual strength

Read spiritual literature

(Bible, *Vedas*, *Bhagavad Gita*, *Koran*, and *Chicken Soup for the Soul* (a series of books), and *The Autobiography of a Yogi* by Swami Parmahansa Yogananda.

Before going forward, test yourself to determine if the material of the chapter is clear.

Test

Now I know that I have healing power.	Y/N
Next time I get sick, I will try to heal myself.	Y/N
There is nothing to lose by trying to heal myself.	Y/N
The more I use my healing power, the better I shall get at it.	Y/N
Real healing happens with self-involvement and faith.	Y/N
I understand that I would not try to heal anyone without the proper education and training.	Y/N

If you have answered yes to most questions, congratulations! However, if you have answered no, there is no need for disappointment. Read this chapter again and again until you are convinced otherwise.

Summary

The next time you get sick, first analyze why you got sick. What can you do to get better? Spend some time in just analyzing that. Study self-help books. You may be spending lot of time reading initially, but with experience each subsequent healing becomes easier and easier. Don't hesitate to seek advice or help, whenever you feel the necessity for it. Get involved in your care physically, mentally, and spiritually. You can also do the following:

Physical level

In acute diseases, increase the rest time, change your diet to soup and toast. But in chronic diseases in addition to the rest time, you also have to eat a balanced, healthy, and alkaline diet in small portions.

Mental level

Increase rest and relaxation time. Read religious scriptures, meet spiritual people, read and study ethical and spiritual values to strengthen the mind. Try to have a total understanding of life as a whole.

Spiritual level

Meditation, read scientific healing affirmations. Make donations to worthy causes or do humanitarian work. Do service to others in any form. Visit temples, churches, synagogues, or mosques.

The key message

We need to create awareness that self-healing is inherent in each one of us. It can be very rewarding. The outcome of self-healing can surpass the results of any other healing method. This is how most great people have healed themselves.

Self-healing is an art and a science. The more you do it, the better you get at it. Every self-healing paves the way for a better subsequent healing. You do not need to have any extensive knowledge, training, or experience to self-heal. You do not need to fear anything. Self-healing builds confidence, strengthens the mind and spirit, and brings joy.

Mantra

I know I have the power to heal myself. In order to enjoy perfect health, I shall keep my body healthy, my mind balanced, and my spirit strong.

CHAPTER FORTY-TWO

Fasting: Cleansing the Body, Mind and Soul

I humbled my soul with fasting.
—*Psalms 69:10*

Fasting cleanses the body, strengthens the mind, and makes the spirit humble. A strong body, mind, and humble spirit are the basis of good health and happiness.

Have you ever thought of living without food for a day or two? There are cases of yogis living without food for a month or so. There is an authentic story of a lady who decided to stop eating after some inner awakening and thereafter she never ate. This story is narrated by Swami Parmahansa Yogananda in his book titled *Autobiography of a Yogi*.

You may be surprised to know that fasting is a very common practice among certain spiritual, religious, and ethnic groups. They use it on a regular basis for the prevention of diseases, maintenance of health, curing of the diseases, building will power, and for spiritual purification. Recently fasting has become a science in itself. Doctors of fasting are known as natural hygienists. These doctors prescribe, supervise, and guide patients during fasting periods. For more information you can contact the American Association of Natural Hygienists.

Objectives

1. Fasting is one of the safest methods not only for prevention of diseases, but also for the treatment of many diseases.

2. Fasting or at least modified fasting can be used by everyone on a regular basis for staying healthy without any fear or danger.

Definition

Fasting is a period of abstinence from food under a controlled environment. Fasting is not starvation. While fasting, you do not need to make any changes in your schedule. You can wake up as usual, go to work as usual, and can even do mild exercises. Heavy exercises during fasting are not recommended. You do not have to worry about proteins and caloric needs, especially if fasting is done over a brief period of time. However, you should meet the daily fluid requirements by taking in adequate amounts of water during fasting. You should avoid tea and coffee. If you are overweight, you can fast as long as 30 to 40 days, but only under the supervision from a physician or someone trained to supervise fasting. However, those people who are accustomed to fasting or fast at periodic intervals can fast without any fear or complication. But people who are not familiar with fasting may need some guidance at least in the beginning.

Misconceptions and clarification

Death

The misconception that people can die of fasting is wrong. Nobody dies of fasting when done under supervision and/or for a brief period of time. Hypoglycemia is also not an issue unless one is underweight or fasting is prolonged.

Water fasting

Water fasting does not mean that one does not drink water; rather it means that one drinks only water. They do not eat or drink anything else except water. Similarly when they are juice fasting, it means that they drink only juices and nothing else.

Milk fasting

Here people drink milk and nothing else for a certain period of time. Milk fasting is common in India. It was done to observe austerity and to gain weight. It was one of the treatment modalities for tuberculosis for patients before the advent of the drugs for tuberculosis.

Fasting an irony

It is strange but true that the best and maximum amount of food is sold during religious fasting. Do you know why? It is also interesting that during the period of fasting, some people think of food more often than during times when they are not fasting.

History

Fasting has been in existence for thousands of years. It is as old a tradition as eating. In olden days no guidance and supervision was available, people used to experiment with their life, and they had the time and patience to do so. Also people who did experiments had better insight and patience. However with the advent of time and research, fasting has become a science.

Dr. Herbert M. Shelton is the pioneer in the field of fasting. His books, *Fasting Can Save Your Life*, *The Science and Fine Art of Fasting*, and *The Pristine Way of Life*, are some of the best books that touch on almost every aspect of fasting. Dr. Joel Fuhrman has written a good book titled *Fasting and Eating for Health*. He has devoted one chapter to the autoimmune disease that is a unique contribution. *Fasting: the Ultimate Diet* by Allen Cot, MD is also worth reading.

Overeating

I'd like to say a few words about overeating. You all know over eating the opposite of fasting; you must have observed yourself, that whenever we study the opposite phenomenon the subject matter becomes clearer. Now let us appreciate the effects of overeating:

1. One often feels heavy, gassy, and gets heartburn. Overeating can cause constipation or diarrhea.

2. One loses an appetite for the next meal, i.e., the time when one feels the need to eat. This creates uneasiness in the mind and the body. For example, if one does not eat one feels weak, but if one eats one gets more bloated.

3. Overeating makes one overweight. Therefore one suffers from the effects of obesity, such as diabetes, high blood pressure, high cholesterol, arthritis, difficulty breathing, heart disease, etc.

4. People who overeat usually require much more sleep versus when they eat normally or in moderate amounts.

5. The over eater has shorter life expectancy. It is well documented in animal experiments that when animals are underfed or fed just right, they live longer, whereas animals that are overfed have shorter life expectancy.

Advantages and disadvantages of fasting

Although fasting has many advantages, everything should be viewed in totality.

Advantages

Fasting helps the person at all levels of the body, mind, and spirit. There should not be any question about it. Even some authors sing laurels in praise of fasting.

Disadvantages

Although fasting is one of the natural healing modalities, if fasting is prolonged and done too often or without supervision, it can cause malnourishment. In later years of life, people who are underweight should not fast without proper guidance unless they are accustomed to it.

How fasting works

Our body is a wonderful dynamic machine that can repair by itself, because of changing dynamics. Fasting provides rest to the digestive system, improves the functioning of the body, and eliminates built-in toxins. When one does not eat, the amount of energy that is used for digestion of the food is diverted for the reparative and healing process. Furthermore, fasting puts the person into anaerobic metabolism for that period, which also has healing effects.

Why people fast (different reasons)

People fast for different purposes. Strangely enough, everybody gets their objectives fulfilled. Following are some of the reasons:

Religious reasons

Many religious, ethnic, and cultural groups fast yearly or semi-annually. It provides social bonding, religious observance, and spiritual cleansing.

Political reasons

In India, Mahatma Gandhi was well known for fasting. He used to fast as many as thirty to forty days at a time to promote his views to the public and to the political leaders.

Spiritual reasons

There is a phrase in the Bible: "I humbled my soul with fasting." Psalms 69:10. Many spiritual leaders observe fasting at regular intervals to observe austerity and to strengthen the body, mind, and soul.

For the sake of sympathy

Some people fast in sympathy, of the suffering of hungry and/or starving people. These people become spiritually strong and connect with cosmic energy.

Fast as a tradition

In India, the fasting tradition is very common among ladies and Indian swamis/gurus. There people fast for the control of the mind and for the purpose of austerity. Austerity makes one strong mentally and spiritually.

Fast for weight loss

This is a popular method, at least in the United States, where fasting is supervised by the natural hygienist.

Fast for an appetite improvement

Here a person fasts whenever he loses the appetite as a result of overeating, e.g., after a party.

Observation of silence

This is known as a "maun fast." During a certain period, e.g., for one, two or three days a person does not speak. This is a time used for reflection of thoughts and for better insight. During this period people are in a spiritual mode and eat only a little vegetarian food.

The experience

Here is a case from my own observation. A sixty-nine-year-old lady came to me with an abdominal obstruction (small bowel), but the obstruction was partial (i.e., not complete). This lady had undergone several surgeries in the past on her abdomen. She was put on a fast and was given IV fluids just to maintain her fluid balance. In a matter of four or five days, she improved, her obstruction disappeared completely, and she regained her normal health.

Many physicians and surgeons must have had similar experiences. Later on I asked this lady how she got sick. She replied that before coming to the hospital, she had been overeating for several days and believed that this was the cause of her condition.

I have also noticed from my personal experience that whenever I fast, I think better, I see better; I hear better, and my body feels lighter. I believe that you can have a similar pleasant experience, if you fast.

Benefits

You can use fasting for multiple purposes. Following is a list that is not complete in any manner, and you can add other benefits from your own experience:

1. Periodic fasting for the maintenance of health.
2. As an adjunct for any chronic treatment modality.
3. To treat all acute (self-limiting) diseases, i.e., colds, coughs, viral, infections, diarrhea
4. To improve or increase appetite
5. People who are underweight can do a milk fast or a modified fast to improve digestion and to have better health.

6. To lose weight

7. To counteract effects of overeating: rest the digestive system for a day or so

8. In most gastrointestinal diseases, observe some modified fasting

9. To provide rest to the digestive system

10. To increase mental acuity

11. To build up will power and strengthen the mind

12. To make oneself humble

Practical points

If you have ever fasted before, you do not need any guidance, and there is no danger. However, if you have never fasted before, proceed as follows:

1. Make a habit of missing one major meal, preferably dinner. Gradually you can build up and learn to skip two consecutive meals in a day. This you can do once or twice a week.

2. Gradually you can extend your fasting up to twenty-four hours without any fear of side effects, if done in this manner.

3. You can do fruit fasting or juice fasting once a week or even two days a week without fear of any side effects or complications, yet with multiple benefits. If you are unfamiliar with this subject, you should read one of the books suggested in this chapter.

4. Short of fasting: If you cannot fast, choose one of the following or any combination thereof:

- Miss one, two, or three meals in a row

- Drink juices for one to three days. Or eat fruit for one to three days in lieu of other food.

- Drink milk or buttermilk for several days. This not only provides adequate nourishment but also puts your stomach to rest and hence improves health.

5. Never overeat: You must be clear from the information presented in this book that fasting has a healing effect, whereas overeating does the opposite. *This is the most important message that you must carry from this chapter.*

It is advisable and important that for the first couple of days after the fast, you should eat light foods; otherwise the positive effects of fasting can be undone. It is also my personal observation.

The key message

Fasting is the cheapest and safest method to provide rest to the digestive system, heal the body, and strengthen the mind. However excessive and prolonged fasting can cause malnourishment and diseases associated with malnourishment. Also one should never overeat. It is better to err on the side of under-eating than overeating.

Mantra

Fasting cleanses the body, strengthens the mind and will power, and humbles the soul. I will miss at least one meal a week to enjoy at least some of the benefits of fasting. I understand that my body is holy. I will respect it and feed it only what is good and healthy after due consideration. In any event I will never overeat.

CHAPTER FORTY-THREE

Hypnotherapy: Healing with Medical Hypnosis

Medical hypnosis is one of the natural healing modalities. It is based upon the fact that in order to change your behavior or mannerism, you need to change or re-program the subconscious mind, because all of your behaviors have their seat in the subconscious mind, and you are the product of good and bad behaviors.

Please also be aware of another useful and practical fact: our mind and subconscious mind are powerful and wonderful elements. These can change, create, recreate, and/or even heal the body.

Objectives

1. With the power of medical hypnosis, you can regain control of your body, mind, and even life.

2. You need to broaden your horizons to the healing power of medical hypnosis/self-hypnosis.

Introduction

Ever since I started using medical hypnosis in my practice, I have seen the practical side of what I always believed. I believe that the mind and the subconscious mind have a profound effect on our body and even on our life.

Definition

According to *The Oxford Dictionary*, hypnosis is the induction of a state of consciousness in which a person loses the power of voluntary action and is highly responsive to suggestions or directions. Hypnosis is a Greek word; *hypno* means sleep, and *osis* means process. However, hypnosis is not sleep. It is a state between sleep and wakefulness. Please be very clear that during the state of medical hypnosis, you are not asleep but are very relaxed.

How medical hypnosis works (heals)

In medical hypnosis the therapist takes the client to a state of deep relaxation or to the level of the subconscious mind. At this level, the client is very open to suggestions. Also one remembers everything that is told to him or her while in the state of hypnosis, thus, life begins to change in accordance with the new suggestions/or programming.

The power of the mind and subconscious mind

Your mind has three states: conscious, subconscious, and super-conscious. In medical hypnosis, we use the power of the subconscious mind.

In the chapter on meditation, I narrated the stories of spiritual masters, who have done wonderful things with the power of their mind and subconscious mind. Some of the stories are narrated in the book titled *Autobiography by a Yogi* by Swami Parmahansa Yogananda. For example:

- A lady saint who never eats
- A saint who never sleeps

- A saint who was buried alive for six weeks and when disinterred, he woke up as if he had been sleeping
- A very old saint, who saw the dead body of a child, collapsed himself purposefully, and then the child woke up. In other words, he transferred his soul from his old body to the body of a deceased child.
- A saint who appeared in two places at the same time

I have witnessed myself the incident of a yogi who stood on the stage and stopped his pulse.

Misconceptions about medical hypnosis

Ignorance breeds fear. It is also equally true that knowledge removes fear. Therefore it is good to remove some misconceptions that may come to your mind before you go for medical hypnosis. Once these fears are removed, you become more open to this modality of treatment.

Q. Can I get stuck in medical hypnosis?

A. No. This does not happen. However on rare occasions, someone may fall asleep. There is no consequence of that. After normal sleep, you will wake up.

Q. Can I be made to do things against my wishes?

A. It is as equally absurd as the first misconception. The job of the hypnotherapist is to help their client. No one can make the client do anything against their wishes, because the client is always in charge and in control.

Q. Is the state of hypnosis something rare or an unusual phenomenon?

A. No. Everybody goes through a state of hypnosis every now and then. Hypnosis is nothing but a state of deep relaxation.

You must have experienced at one time or another that you are sitting and relaxing on a beach or in your own backyard for hours, and suddenly you realize that so much time has passed away. It is all because you were so relaxed or sort of in the state of hypnosis.

You may have also occasionally experienced that you go from one place to another without realizing how you got there. It did not matter whether you were driving or walking. It is again because all this time you were in state of deep relaxation or hypnosis.

Medical hypnosis vs. stage hypnosis

Medical hypnosis and stage hypnosis are two separate entities. In stage hypnosis, the hypnotic selects the most vulnerable person and makes them do things for the sake of fun and enjoyment of the audience. But in medical hypnosis, the hypnotherapist is focused only on healing the client. The client is not vulnerable and is in full control. Also the hypnotic session can be terminated easily at any time, at the will and desire of the subject, as well as by the hypnotherapist.

Key message

1. People should be open to explore medical hypnosis as a healing modality.
2. Anybody can learn and use self-hypnosis for building confidence, to build mind power and to get back the control of their life.

Mantra

My life and I are the direct products of my mind and the subconscious mind. With the power of medical hypnosis and self-hypnosis, I can bring about the desired changes in the subconscious mind and hence in my life.

Till Next Time

(*Namastee*)

This is my first book. Writing this book was a very enriching and rewarding experience for me. I have seen my life transform as I was writing each chapter.

I hope you have enjoyed reading this book, and that it was an educational and an enriching experience for you. I hope it has brought some inner awakening or that your third eye has opened, or your sixth sense has been activated. I would like to think that you have made some positive changes in your life already. I am also sure that today you must think and feel differently about yourself than you ever did before in your life.

It must be clear to you by now that you are complete and whole, and you have huge potential. You do not need to depend upon anything or anyone else, at least for your health and happiness. You have it all. This message must have brought a deep level of satisfaction, joy, and happiness. You must feel free and liberated. What a great feeling! You must have also come to another realization, that if you want longevity, health, and happiness in life, you have to take responsibility for every act and outcome, good or bad. This is the only way.

I also believe that whatever benefits you have obtained from the first reading of this book, you can continue to add a little extra with each subsequent reading or re-reading, because I have covered a vast amount of information, and it is difficult to grasp all the information in one reading.

I sincerely believe that if you choose even one message from every chapter/poem/mantra and act upon it , it could change your life.

I would like you to ask you a final and sincere question: Do you feel younger, healthier, and happier now than before you read this book? If so, why not help others by spreading or sharing this message? You can do it in millions of ways. You could give this book to a friend, a dear one, or to your local library, or you could persuade your local librarian to make this book available for the general public. This book should make a perfect gift for any occasion, for example, a birthday, wedding anniversary, Christmas, Valentine's Day, etc. If you are a health professional or any other professional, you could have a copy in your reception room or waiting area.

I would like to thank you once again for giving me the opportunity to be part of your health and happiness. I wish you good luck!

Pratap C. Singhal, MD

Appendix A: Poems

I have expressed some of the salient points of the following chapters in the form of poetry. I have done this because poems have deeper and longer-lasting effects on one's mind and soul. These poems appear at the end of several chapters. I have listed some of them on this page for people who enjoy poetry.

1. Introduction: I am the master of my domain
2. Dynamics of health: In life everything is on the go: It could be fast or slow
3. Balance: Balance is the secret of everything
4. Energy: Energy is immortal, so is everything
5. Who am I? Part 1: Understanding self is the game of its own kind
6. Who am I? Part 2: Let us go home
7. Definition of health: What is health?
8. Digestion: When food becomes health
9. Ego: 1. I am no body, no body
   2. Hero and zero is the game of life
10. Intelligence: Pain and suffering belongs to the unwise, freedom and happiness is the symbol of the wise
11. Mind: A. Life is a game, it is the game of the mind
    B. Please make up your mind, make up.
12. Soul: How could I ever die, this is a great surprise

13. Spirituality: My friend it is a secret of life

14. Sleep: Rise and awake

15. Silence: Silence is everywhere and in everything

16. God: 1. Oh God grant me the wisdom so that I can enjoy the life of happiness and freedom.

    2. Whom to fear and what to fear

17. Happiness: Life is game, If one plays it right it shall be a happy game

18. Young forever: I am always young, because my mind is young

Glossary

A

Arjuna – A warrior in Mahabharta, a Vedic scholar, and pupil of Lord Krishna

Ayurveda – The most ancient healing medical science that originated from India

Allopathy – The conventional medical healing science, based upon the laws of contraries, whereas homeopathy is based upon the laws of similar

B

Bhagavad Gita – A treatise, the summary of the metaphysical science as sung by Lord Krishna, (also a chapter in Yajurveda). After reading this scripture, the fear of death goes away

Bhai – Brother in Hindi language

Bible – Christian scripture consisting of Old and New testaments, the Jewish scripture consists of Torah or law, the prophets and the Hagiographa or writing

C

Cure – Healing means becoming whole or complete, returning to normal health

D

Disease – Dis+ease, not at ease or discomfort

Dayanand Swami – (February 12, 1824 – October 31, 1883) A great yogi, a swami, a Vedic scholar, and a social reformer of his time. Also the transcriber of the Vedas in simple, plain, understandable language for the average person

E

Ether – The clear sky, the upper region beyond the clouds, a substance formally postulated to permeate all spaces and transmit light; also one of the first and most primitive forces that leads to the formation of atom (the first physical element of the universe). In sequence: ether→ air→ fire→ water→atom

Eternal – Lasting or existing forever, essentially unchanged, for example God, nature, or souls

F

Fast – Absence from food with a purpose for certain duration, not starvation

G

Guru – Hindu spiritual teacher, also each of the ten first leaders of Sikh religion

H

Health – Sound physical and mental health

Happiness – Sound physical and mental health, plus contentment and adeptness

Homeopathy – A medical healing art and science 200 years old, founded by Hahnemann and originated in Germany, based upon the laws of similar, whereas allopathy is based upon the laws of contraries.

I

Immortal – Living forever, deserving to be remembered forever

K

Koran – Islamic sacred book, believed to be the word of God, as dictated to Mohammad and written in Arabic

Krishna or Lord Krishna – A guru, a yogi in Mahabharata, believed to be incarnation of deity Vishnu by some Hindus

M

Mahabharata – One of the greatest epics of India, depicting a story between the prince (Kaurava) and his cousin brothers (Pandavas) based on the right and wrong

Meditator – A person who practice meditation on a regular basis

Meta physics – *Meta*, means beyond, *physical* means body; meta denotes something of a higher order

Monk – Member of religious community of men living under vows of poverty, chastity and obedience

Mantra – Originally in Hinduism and Buddhism, a word or sound repeated to aid concentration in meditation; or a statement or slogan repeated frequently for the benefit of the mind

R

Rama or Lord Rama – Believed to be the reincarnation of God by some Hindus

Rishi – A Hindu sage or saint

Rig-Veda – As defined by *The Oxford Dictionary*, the oldest principle of Vedas. From Sanskrit Rig-Veda means sacred *stanga*. Also the first and the oldest book listed in the Library of Congress with prose/mantras

Reincarnation – Rebirth of a soul into a new body

S

Saint – A person acknowledged as holy or virtuous

Sanskara – A purifactory ceremony or rite making a major event in one's life; means making perfect preparations

Swami – A male Hindu religious teacher

Sudama – One of the religious person, a classmate, and a friend of Lord Krishna.

U

Upanishad – Each of the series of Hindu sacred treatises written in Sanskrit expounding the Veda in reference to God, soul and the meta physical body; in Sanskrit it means to sit near

V

Veda – The most ancient Hindu scriptures, four in number, namely with Rig Veda, Yajur Veda, Sam Veda, and Athar Veda. Veda also means knowledge or book of knowledge.

Vivekanand, Swami – (1853-1902) A great Indian philosopher and teacher of metaphysical science, who traveled the USA and abroad. He devoted his life to this mission.

Y

Yudhistra – One of the five main characters of Mahabharata. Vedic and religious scholar and a warrior

Yama – In Hindu belief, Yama is the king of the dead and death, who controls death.

Index

BOOK AVAILABILTY

This book is available everywhere you can contact any of the following:

1. The author, Pratap C. Singhal MD

   431 Washington Avenue, Belleville, NJ USA 07109

   Phone: 1-973-759-2241

   go to his website: www.livehealthierlivehappier.com
2. The publisher: www.wastelandpress.net
3. Amazon.com
4. Barnes and Noble
5. Books-a-Million
6. and many other retailers worldwide...

Bibliography

Section A: Spiritual

- Art of Happiness: His Holiness The Dalai Lama, Narrated by Howard Cutler MD
- Why God permits Evil and How to rise above it: Paramahansa Yogananda
- Living Fearlessly: Paramahansa Yogananda
- Metaphysical Meditation: Paramahansa Yogananda
- Autobiography of a Yogi: Paramahansa Yogananda
- Intuition Soul guide for life decisions: Sri Daya Mata
- Spiritual Teaching of Hinduism Veda Niketan Publication: Nardev Vedalamkar
- Hindu Satakam: Deen Bandhu Chandora Sharma
- Complete work of Swami Vivekanand
- Introduction to Veda: Swami Dayanand
- Light of truth: Swami Dayanand
- Bhagwad Geeta, as narrated by Lord Krishna
- Scientific Healing Affirmations - Paramahansa Yogananda
- Vedic Philosophy- teaching of Hinduism

- **Section B: Physical**
- Fit for Life : Harvey & Marilyn Diamond
- Macrobiotic Path to total Health: Michio Kushi & Alex Jack

- Fasting can save your life: Herbert M. Sheltion Published by American Natural Hygiene Society.
- Fasting the Ultimate Diet: Allan Cott
- Fasting and eating for health: Dr. Joel Fulhrmann
- Food that heals natural way to good health: H. K. Bakhru MD
- Food is your best medicine: Henry G. Bieler MD
- Total fitness in 30 minutes a week: Dr. Laurence E. Morehouse Phd & Leonard Gross
- Healthy Healing, An alternative healing reference: Linda G. Rector Page, N.D. PhD
- Prescription for nutritional healing: James F. Balch MD and Phyllis A. Balch CNC.
- Nutrition Almanac Third Edition: Lavon J. Dunne

- **Section C: General**
- Complete System of Self-Healing, The internal exercises: Stephen T. Chang
- Edgar Cayce Handbook for health through drugless therapy: Harold J. Reilly & Ruth Hagy Brod. A.R.E (Association of Research and Enlightenment) Virginia Beach, Virginia
- Education and the Significance of Life: Dr. Krishnamurti
- Art of Life : Ritu Chopra
- How to argue and win everytime, at home, at work, in court, everywhere and every day, Gerry Spence
- Hinduism time
- Excerpts from the Fundamentals of Maharishi Ayurveda prepared by Richard Acerbach, MD., F.A.A.F.P. and Stuart Rothenberg, MD., F.A.A.F.P.

- Alkalize or die. By Dr. Theodore Abroody
- Cure of common diseases. By Dr. Vithaldas Modi

Breinigsville, PA USA
08 October 2010
246956BV00003B/4/P

9 781600 474132